Let's E.A.T!

Break the addictive cycle of dieting,
lose weight and make peace with food
and your body... for life.

Lisa Carpenter, CNC, CSNC,
PN1, CPT

Photography credits to:
Meigan Canfield Photography (front cover)
Sandra Steier (back cover)

ISBN-10: 1981430881

ISBN-13: 978-1981430888

CONTENTS

Dedication

Writing a book was a dream that found me thanks to the encouragement of my family, coaches, mentors, clients, colleagues and friends. I'm forever grateful for the people in my life who've challenged me to shine brighter and step into a bigger vision for myself and my business. Each of you hold a special place in my heart.

I wouldn't be who I am or where I am today without the guidance, support and love from each of you and the universal magic and faith that guides my life.

To my beautiful boys Colton, Logan and Jake.

You are the reason I dream big. May you always have the courage to go after the lives you want and the belief in yourself to achieve your heart's deepest desires.

To the man I share my life with.

I love you. I wouldn't change a single thing, and I am grateful for all of it.

To my parents.

Thank you for all the ways you show me love and support my dreams. I didn't always make it easy for you, and I'm grateful for the relationship we have today. All of this is possible because you welcomed me into the world and into your hearts. I'm grateful for both of you.

To Joshua.

You brought my vision to life and because of you, my work will impact lives around the world. Thank you for your magic.

XO ~ Lisa

Resources

Understanding the relationship between your feelings and food does not end here!

Go to LisaCarpenter.ca/Book for resources such as:

- The Feelings Wheel
- H.A.L.T! & P.A.I.N. Printable Reminders
- The Ultimate List of Codependent Behaviours (And How to Avoid Them)
- Suggested Daily Mantras
- SOS Audio Downloads

...and much, much more!

Introduction

You've been down this road before. Every time you find yourself here, you promise yourself it will be different.

This time, is the last time.

This familiar journey starts with an early morning weigh in, chicken and salad for lunch with a side of vegetables and some sort of green protein smoothie filled with "healthy" stuff that looks (and tastes) like swamp.

What a reward for that 3 hour fat-burning cardio session.

Inevitably, this journey soon ends with the scale in the trash, salads replaced by takeout pizza (with double cheese) and a pop in your hand while Googling "body positive articles."

If the past 3 paragraphs have described your struggle with nutrition and weight loss to the "T", then you've come to the right place.

I wrote this book for you -- yes, *YOU* -- because there is a problem in our social consciousness when it comes to all things food and health.

Since 1985, obesity rates have *tripled*. In North America, we've gone from 1 in 15 adults with a Body Mass Index (BMI) that makes the cardiologist cringe to 1 in 5.

Of course, we can blame everything from greasy fast food to carb-rich fad diets, but these are symptoms, *not the problem itself.*

Over the last 30 years, while every health guru and workout junkie has been scolding us for sneaking a handful of chocolate chips before bedtime, spending on health and wellness products has exploded, from a few billion dollars a year to over *3 trillion.*

Why should you care about this?

Because data doesn't lie. And this particular data tells us a truth more uncomfortable than a sweat-drenched scratchy cotton sweater after an evening at the gym.

The more we've spent on our health as a society, the unhealthier we've become.

Re-read that a few times if you have to. Until it sinks in.

Whether you were aware of this insane correlation or not, you picked up this book for a reason.

This is the last time.

But you'll keep reading it for a very different one. You'll see why in a moment.

While everyone following mainstream advice is focused on seeing the numbers drop -- pounds, inches, etc. -- I'm over here waving my arms like a madwoman trying to draw people's attention to the most important pieces of the puzzle they've been missing.

Amidst our hustle to obey the newest tummy-trimming fad featured on the cover of *Woman's Day*, what if we've been asking ourselves the wrong questions?

What if *that* explains the ironic relationship we have with our Weight Watchers subscription and why we starve ourselves all day of "weigh in" only to gobble down a tub of Ben & Jerry's after? (Because, you know you've saved your points, right?!)

And when the accountability is gone, so is our desire to count points.

Hello, weight gain.

What if losing weight isn't about weight loss?

What if falling in love with your body has nothing to do with changing it?

And what if enjoying your favorite foods doesn't mean you should deprive yourself the rest of the time?

These aren't rhetorical questions; this is my worldview.

It's why people like my client Carlie come to me with skepticism but leave feeling beautiful and empowered -- all after implementing the E.A.T! Framework.

"Not only did my body change, but my thinking about food and body image did too," Carlie told me. "Thank you for helping me feel beautiful again."

I believe this book needs to exist because we've been lied to.

We've been led to believe that a healthy future is someone else's responsibility -- usually some 6-packed, airbrushed Expert-of-the-Month, whose revolutionary new diet plan promises to slice pounds off your thighs like a knife through butter.

From promises of "10 inches gone in 10 days flat" to "better eating, better sex," these gurus offer clickbait as satisfying as a buffet of iceberg lettuce.

So, why does it work?

Because we're looking for that someone with an easy, quick fix -- the fastest solution from point A to B to save us from ourselves and the constant emotional pain we're in. In the process, the food gurus end up doing more harm than good by perpetuating body shame and guilt in the name of accountability. We deprive ourselves of what our bodies need to thrive. We *disempower* ourselves.

And eventually, they break us.

Week after week, I listen to the stories of new clients who recite every mistake they've already made. Blaming and shaming themselves, all they seem to know how to do, is fail (their words).

"It's just so HARD!"

Of course it is!

When we abuse ourselves emotionally, *of course* weight loss will be stiflingly difficult. It would be like trying to train an animal by yelling insults at her. The more intense you are, the less the animal would want to cooperate.

An abused animal bites back.

It's the same with our bodies.

Let's change that. *Forever.*

I want every woman to find her confidence, live a life of abundance, exercise self-control lovingly and ·· most importantly ·· *empower herself.* So what you'll find in the following pages is not a finger-wagger who assigns a grade to every piece of food and sip of beverage that enters your mouth. What *you* eat has no effect on the size of *my* ass.

You're going to learn how to be in the driver's seat of your choices. Not because you've been told what to eat, but because you'll understand what "choice" truly means.

Most diets use shame to motivate us because we have this harmful belief that feeling bad about ourselves will make us behave better.

Not me.

Not this book.

In fact, that very belief is keeping you stuck from breaking free from the diet roller coaster.

The Framework you'll dig into here works because it is *not* based on developing the rugged self-discipline of a soldier so you can post a jaw-dropping before-and-after photo on social media.

Let me tell you a secret -- *There is no after!*

Think about it. When will there be a time in your life "after" you're done choosing what foods to put in your body, when you're done moving your body in a way that feels good, when you're done enjoying the kind of energy you've always desired?

There is no after.

Dieting perpetuates the belief that when we get "there," we'll be done. With a poof of fairy dust, we'll magically love and accept our bodies when the weight is gone. Then we'll no longer have to be mindful of our choices.

This simply isn't how it works in the real world.

If you start a business, you don't quit after making a million bucks. That kind of a milestone is inspiration to keep going, to stay the course.

So there is no after. Tattoo that onto the back of your hand, if you have to.

Instead, I'm going to teach you a Framework to help you create a mindset and lifestyle around food and your body. It'll become a habit, just like brushing your teeth is already.

In the mad rush to change the way we look, we often miss the entire point of eating well.

Whether you want to consistently embrace the right nutrition to improve your health overall, or right now you're just trying to lose a few inches and drop the weight that's keeping you out of your favourite outfit, this is primarily an *emotional* journey we're on together. It seems Other People's Advice very rarely mentions this.

It's easy (and cheap) to shove a diet plan PDF into your face; it's much, *much* harder to hold space for someone who wants to take back control of her life and choices.

If you know anything about my work as a Transformational Life and Nutrition Coach, you know I thrive on the latter.

Together, we'll acknowledge the teeth-grinding, tear-jerking emotions that play a role in eating well, losing weight and regaining your energy and confidence.

So while everyone else is looking for a guarantee that <insert new fad> will absolutely-and-with-no-questions-asked make you lose X pounds per day over the next 4 weeks, you can step outside the matrix of shame and guilt to apply principles that actually work.

And the best part? YOU make the rules, and YOU set the pace right from the get-go.

One of my favorites that I share with clients is an old cliche told with a fresh interpretation: *How do you eat an elephant? One bite at a time.*

That means looking at every single meal you eat. Being aware of and then appreciating what you did with those meals and your nutritional choices.

Celebrate the hell out of every conscious choice you make, then move on to the next meal. No guilt, no shame, and no judgment while taking 100% ownership and responsibility for your choice.

Doesn't that sound freeing?

The E.A.T! Framework is actually based on this process, so you will be learning and applying it in several layers.

Learn one layer at your own pace, apply it without judgment or guilt and move on to the next one when you're ready.

Rather than have me tell you what to eat or what not to -- that is no one's responsibility but yours -- I will show you how to first *feel empowered* to make the right choices for you (Chapters 1-8). Then once you understand what it means to have a relationship with food, I'll show you how to *make* those choices within the Framework (Chapters 9-15).

This may feel like a lot. But it's not. *Really.*

There is no such thing as perfection, only progress.

Progress is the domain of emotional healing.

After learning how to make choices that felt right for her within the E.A.T! Framework, my client Michelle told me, "I have come to know a person I didn't know existed. I can look in the mirror and see the authentic me staring back."

Since 2003, I've dreamed of creating a world full of Michelle's, where no woman has to look outside of herself to make the right choices. Learn a proven Framework, and personalize the hell out of it so you can look the way you want to look and feel the way you want to feel. That's why I devote an entire section of this book to just your *relationship* with food!

And notice I didn't say in the last paragraph, ". . .so you can *achieve your goals.*"

Stop playing the losing game everyone else is, where you idolize a number that remains just out of reach, no matter how much guilt you wallow in or how much you punish yourself. Besides, any number only means something because you've decided it does. The number on the scale is only a reflection of your relationship with gravity. Nothing more, nothing less.

It doesn't reflect your self worth, your value as a human being, how much you love and are loved or the impact you're having in this world.

Your worth is not your weight.

Please let that sink in for just a moment.

After your read this book -- not "finish" it -- and learn the E.A.T! Framework, my hope is that you will hurry over to Amazon.com to pen a review with the thrill of a toddler on Christmas morning surrounded by unwrapped gifts.

My prayer is that your experience with me between these pages will be so much more than pounds and inches lost -- you'll feel like a new person.

Because you'll *be* one. The one you've always wanted to become but never quite knew how -- or how to stay the course.

My client Jennifer shared an insight after going from hiding behind a wardrobe several sizes too large, to toning her physique and looking like a fitness model.

"I learned to take back control of me and my choices for healthy eating and not to deprive myself. Now I take the time and make better choices about what I put into my body."

Better choices, better outcomes.

In her case, everyone looks at her outward transformation with awe, jealousy or lust. Or all three. Yes, she applied my framework to fit her needs, but all progress started with her relationship with food.

Change that, and you change everything else.

In a world where every yo-yo dieter screams, "Just give me a plan! Just tell me what to do!" let's focus first on the emotions surrounding your eating habits.

Ever heard of the 80/20 Rule? It basically states that 80% of your outcomes are a result of only 20% of your total effort.

Understanding your relationship with food is that 20%. Without it, even the E.A.T! Framework will be an endless struggle.

I can speak and write so confidently about this because this feedback comes to me every single day! Not too long ago, a physician near my hometown shared with me, "I am changing my relationship with food and as a result improving my health and my body."

As a result -- this simple phrase is the ticket to a lifetime of body confidence, nutritious meals and endless energy.

With this book, I humbly offer you that ticket.

So don't skip ahead to the last page to see how the book "ends." And don't take yourself too seriously. We're on this journey together, and I promise that if you allow yourself to become empowered, it will be *easy* to lose whatever weight or inches have haunted your figure for months, years or even decades.

We'll get there.

One bite at a time.

PROGRESS NOT PERFECTION

At the close of every chapter, you will have the opportunity to bring what you learn to life -- immediately. But the lessons don't end between these pages!

To get free instant access to worksheets, resources and downloads that make this book even easier to implement, visit LisaCarpenter.ca/Book.

Chapter 1
The Last Diet Book You'll Ever Need

If the only thing that happens for you after reading this book is dropping a few pounds, I failed.

Losing weight is easy, even my clients know this. After all, you have probably lost weight many, MANY times.

Eating healthy isn't rocket science either. Everyone knows the importance of moving their bodies.

But if it was as easy as calories in versus calories out, we'd all be fit and healthy.

For every step of progress, most women I work with find themselves taking 2 steps backward.

With every diet program out there, we get lost in a sea of rules, our confidence sinking in a losing battle.

You do well for awhile, but when stress hits, you hit the cupboard for the chips and cookies. Then the in-stant gratification gives way to sustained guilt because you "failed."

And there you are, stuck on a carousel that never stops turning.

Losing the weight and watching it sneak back onto our bodies again can make diets feel like pure hell.

Like the Garfield comic strip tells us, "Diet is 'die' with a 't.'"

So to clarify my opening statement, I want so much more for you than a one-time goal achieved. I want this to be the last diet book you ever read because the days of *needing* to hop on and hop off a self-depriving plan are over.

For good.

Forever.

I take the stand that total transformation comes not from losing the weight, but what happens *before* the pounds are shed and the inches are lost.

A perfect example of how the E.A.T! Framework does this is Keri-Anne's story:

"What is it about working with you, Lisa Carpenter? I have done weight loss and weight gain but something so much deeper is here today -- three years later. And that is honouring my body in a new way. To feel like a partner with my body -- engaged, connected, proud and lovingly responsible for the experience I have in this vehicle of my dreams. This is what you and your program offer -- not just weight loss. That shit is one dimensional and frankly, easy. I can do my way through weight loss. But being in weight loss is an entirely different deal -- and you get this. It's the living in and partnering with my body is what I'm getting now. I'm so grateful for finally feeling inspired and fuelled."

Keri-Anne never has to diet again. Neither will you.

And while you're at it, why not just take that word completely out of your vocabulary?

"Healthy."

The convergence of fad diets and targeted advertising have completely distorted its definition.

It all starts with the food manufacturers and their marketing departments, whose goal is to push our hot buttons to get us to buy.

That's all they care about. That's what they're after.

Not to help us lose weight. Not to make us feel good about ourselves. Not to empower us to love ourselves.

Not a day goes by without you hearing something about nutrition. And it's usually someone with absolutely ZERO expertise in nutrition (they do have a super-sized PR budget though).

A few months ago, such a person mouthed off over the radio airwaves. The claim?

"A small can of Coke everyday can actually be a healthy treat for you."

Turns out, this self-proclaimed nutritionist was an employee of the Coca-Cola Company. Big surprise!

This isn't about me bashing Coke or telling you that Coke isn't healthy for you. As we dive into the E.A.T! Framework, you'll find that I don't put judgments on food as being "good" or "bad." Those words are the language of guilt, shame and judgment.

The point is, it's up to you to be discerning about what you do or don't put into your body.

That's why E.A.T! is a Framework -- a framework is a basic structure that can be modified as needed.

So you don't blindly follow what some food manufacturer or guru tells you is healthy for you. What works for you comes down to YOUR individual choice.

It's about time we start eating for ourselves rather than eating what someone else tells us to. There is no one-diet-fits-all eating plan.

Not low-fat, no-carb, paleo, or gluten-free.

In the days of big hair, disco and poorly acted exercise videotapes, the low-fat diets were the rage.

"Get rid of fats! Go fat-free! Throw away your butter!"

Fat is incredibly calorically dense -- 9 calories per gram -- whereas proteins and carbohydrates have only 4.

So the belief was, if we removed fats from our food, we'd see a radical drop in caloric intake and everybody would lose weight and suddenly become healthy.

Literally the opposite happened. Fat makes food taste good, and it helps us feel full and satisfied. So when fat disappeared from staple foods, there was no "off button" for eating.

We kept eating more and more carbohydrates to satisfy our appetites. To make newly bland foods taste good again, manufacturers dumped real and artificial sweeteners into everything. Sweet makes us crave sweet, so calorie over-consumption exploded.

Those low-fat diets didn't fix the obesity problem, they accelerated it. Then popular culture moved on to the low- and no-carbohydrate diets, thinking "Okay, so fat isn't the problem. It must be the carbs!"

Here's the thing about carbohydrates; not all carbs are created equal (Chapter 11). As gasoline is to a car, so carbohydrates are to the body.

In other words, carbs are the official energy food of human beings. So there's no good reason to remove them from our meal plans outright. Instead, let's be respectful of the role they play.

But is that what most people do?

No. Most people either consume carbs like they're training for an Ironman competition or avoid them like the plague. So to keep our carb intake sane, we need to stop fearing them and learn which ones are best for our bodies. E.A.T! has you covered. The next time you see any diet telling you to eliminate an entire macronutrient, you have permission to be completely suspicious of it.

After the low-carb, no-carb, slow-carb phase came paleo. I'll have to tread lightly here because many of my clients come to me while on the paleo diet, and I am on board with aspects of it.

For instance, I do love that paleo is all about foods from the earth. However, not all of us need to cut out grains.

My critique applies to the gluten-free fad as well. Instead of painting an entire food group with a broad brushstroke, pay attention to how different foods make you feel. THEN decide what you want to eat and what you don't. Learn to listen to your body, and let it and your intuition guide you.

So if grains upset your stomach, don't eat them. If they don't (and you enjoy them), why would you take them out? Because somebody else told you a grain-free diet is the fastest path to weight loss? I call BS.

That is NOT empowering, especially since the right kind of grains can be a powerful food group to help you feel your best (Chapter 11).

Remember, lead, uranium and cocaine are all gluten-free, too! Beware of health buzzwords. Only YOU can determine what foods make you feel, look and perform your best.

And I'll help you get there. Note that the "how" of my E.A.T! framework doesn't come until Chapter 9 for a reason. The "why" must come first. Expecting you to blindly follow yet another nutrition program would be hypocritical.

Like Keri-Ann, you'll get educated and empowered *first* so you can step back and really determine what's best for you.

I want you to OWN that responsibility. YOU call the shots about your body, damn it! There is NOTHING wrong with you.

Imagine no longer believing that you're broken and need fixing.

There is also nothing wrong with wanting to lose weight -- unless your motivation is built on the belief that you are not good enough as you are right now. Weight loss won't make you feel better unless you start to feel better about yourself right now as you are.

Embrace who you need to be, yes. That does mean changing who you are right now, but shame and blame cannot be part of that progress. There's nothing wrong with who you are right now. The journey is the destination.

That message won't sell diet pills, so you will NEVER hear it from the industry.

The popular dieting cycle, whether it's low-fat or low-carb, focuses instead on "fixing" yourself as fast as possible. That's why it keeps us stuck for *years*.

The graph below offers a visual of what I mean.

We get into a diet, we're all in, we work our little buns off, and we follow the plan.

High intensity in a short amount of time.

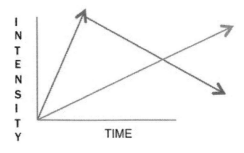

Then what happens?

We can only maintain that level of intensity and will-power for a short time. When it diminishes, so do our motivation and momentum.

Pretty soon, we end up right back where we started -- or worse.

Back to the elephant metaphors, there's an expression that asks, "How long can you steer an elephant for?"

If you've ever seen an elephant, the answer will be obvious -- *not very long!*

Eventually, that elephant is going to win because it's going to overpower you.

The same goes for eating right and living well. Fast and furious never works; I prefer steady and methodical because it *does*.

This is the difference between lovingly building supportive habits versus punishing ourselves with boring workouts and food we hate.

Yes, it is possible to build those habits without depriving yourself! I can give you the resources you need -- and I do just that in the chapters ahead -- but it will require you to *become who you want to be*.

You'll learn to make different choices one at a time, from your inner dialogue to meal planning. It's not easy, but I promise it's different from anything you've ever tried before.

As you take baby steps along the way, you'll look at food differently. That new perspective is the foundation to create new habits.

I've had women take one look at that diet graph and burst into uncontrollable tears.

"That's it! That's why I keep failing!"

The all-in, head-down, get-her-done attitude right out of the gate cannot work. New habits are not made in a day.

If you really do want to create a lifestyle for the long-term, you must pace yourself. This means slowing the process down. It means doing less, *better*. It means focusing on progress, not perfection, and allowing the journey to be part of the destination.

Like I explained in the Introduction, there's no place to get to, there's no "after" because a lifestyle is never done. It becomes who you are, shapes what you do and creates results that stay with you indefinitely.

But with a diet, you get on it, hit your weight loss goals and off you go. Then the cycle starts all over again. It's exhausting, defeating and feeds all sorts of self defeating beliefs playing in your subconscious mind.

Repeat after me, "NO. MORE. DIETS."

Only YOU can take radical responsibility for how your body looks and feels. No one else can get you the results you want. No diet, no coach, no specially designed meal plan. You've got to be the one who gets back into the driver's seat of your choices.

But if we don't take responsibility for our circumstances, release our need to blame previous diets and continue to feel like crap, we become victims of ourselves. We learn helplessness and forget we've had the power all along.

So your approach to weight loss should not be to obey a plan -- not even mine!

What do *you* want out of weight loss?

Really.

There is no "right" objective here.

Maybe you're tired of commiserating with friends behind closed doors about how many junk food snacks you had at work last week.

Maybe you're just OVER the emotion of feeling perpetually sad. It sucks to have zero confidence in public, I get it.

Maybe you're sick of not fitting into clothes, of not showing up in the world the way you want to, of hiding behind others whenever there's a spontaneous photo shoot with family or friends.

If that's the case, a lightbulb probably came on when you read that first perspective-altering question in the Introduction.

"What if losing weight isn't about weight loss?"

That was EXACTLY the case for my client Cathy. For her -- and for millions of women like her -- weight loss isn't about losing weight, it's about being free to *live life to the fullest.*

"I finally have the energy that I was lacking. I couldn't remember what it was like to actually feel like doing stuff instead of being tired all the time. I have lost a few more pounds and a few inches but most importantly, I am feeling like a participant in life instead of an observer!"

Having a body-positive attitude doesn't mean we blindfold ourselves when it comes to size, weight or overall health. Of course I don't believe in fat-shaming. Staring into every mirror and quietly uttering profanities at yourself gets nobody anywhere.

On the other hand, the body positive movement is not an excuse to give up on our health -- it's a reason to LOVE our bodies, CHERISH nutritious food and MAKE empowering decisions.

By reading this book, you're telling the Universe that you're ready to have *eating* become an act of self-love. Food is no longer a weapon of abuse and dieting torture.

As with any habit changes, lasting results don't come from rigid rules or immediate intensity at the start.

In fact, transformation doesn't come from what you *do*, it's about *who you become*.

So let me ask you:

Who do you need to become to get lasting results?

Who do you need to become to lose weight with ease?

Who do you need to become to embrace a healthy lifestyle and ditch dieting?

Who would you be if you gave up your addiction to dieting?

When I walk clients through the process of answering these questions in *Feelings & Food*, I explain that your answers should read like a story.

Imagine your future self.

What would your life be like?

How would things change?

What would be different?

How do you feel in your new life?

Then get really specific.

What would you be wearing, what activities would you be participating in, what would the relationship with your partner, kids, family and your body look like?

How would you feel when you get up in the morning and go to bed at night? What would your relationship with food look like?

Pretend you have a magic wand and conjure that perfect picture without holding back any details or dreaming small. A journal is the ideal place to start writing your answers. Allow your imagination whisk you away into the life of future you.

However detailed or simple your story is, keep it handy. Re-read it daily. This will become your new reality as you start making choices in alignment with it. As Walt Disney told us, "If you can dream it, you can do it."

Walt Disney is the perfect example of a dreamer who refused to give up. He saw his future so clearly that even after his first animation company's bankruptcy and a rumored 302 "No's" for financing, he kept moving forward. His Why -- and his imagination -- created the magic of Disney World that we now all know and love.

Can you imagine no Mickey, Donald or Magic Kingdom?

Like Walt Disney, your success starts with you allowing yourself to see it, feel it and believe in it. . .*before* it has manifested.

An ambition without a vision is like Christmas morning without any presents. All thrill, no substance.

Imagine if Walt had accepted all those "No's" and labelled himself a failure. Instead, he decided to not let his bankruptcy or inability to get financing define him. He kept trying -- for the love of his Why. He wanted to create a place where children and their parents could have fun together. He mapped out every detail and kept progressing until his vision was realized. He grew into the CEO, visionary and successful entrepreneur he needed to become.

Your vision for your body's future is no different. As I explained at the beginning of this chapter, the truth is, it's really not about the weight. Becoming the person you've always hoped you could be is about asking yourself the questions, "What do you want, and why do you want it?"

If you know why you want to lose that weight and why you want to have a better relationship with food and your body, what would change for you?

What would change when you get there?

How will you feel?

What kind of things will you be doing?

Spend time with these questions and journal your answers. In case you don't have a journal, I've included space at the end of this chapter to let your mind be free on paper. Just thinking about them isn't enough. You must write them out for your unconscious beliefs to surface.

Be as specific as possible. Get very clear on what you want. Then keep going deeper, asking yourself, "But *why* do I want that? And why do I want *that?*"

Why is such an important question that we cannot afford to only ask it once. So this is not meant to be a surface level exercise you glance at and think, "Oh, that's nice," then move on to the next chapter without even attempting it.

Let yourself go deeper than you ever have.

Keep digging.

Your Why will guide your journey. You must connect to it beyond the surface stuff like fitting into skinny jeans or just feeling more confident.

Chart your course to the future you desire, and you'll get there. I promise.

PROGRESS NOT PERFECTION

Define your goals and understand why you want to achieve them *for you* -- not for anyone else.

In the space provided, answer this strategic series of questions. Don't skip them. It might be tough to get through it, but it WILL pay off in the end.

---

1. What Do you Want?

Is This Really About You?

2. What Do you Want?

Is This Really About You?

3. What **Do** you **Want?**

Is This Really About You?

4. What **Do you Want?**

Is This Really About You?

---

1. Why **Do you Want it?**

2. Why **Do you Want it?**

3. Why **Do you Want it?**

4. Why **Do you Want it?**

5. Why **Do you Want it?**

Chapter 2
Feelings and Food

"Emotional eating."

Anyone who's ever struggled with weight gain, overeating, yo-yo diets or a lack of self esteem knows those 2 words well.

You feel like shit, you eat. You had a bad day, you eat. You're bored at night, you eat. You just want to feel something good before bed, you eat.

It happens.

So does the guilt.

I bet nobody's told you *why* emotional eating is a thing though. In fact, this might be the first time you're putting 2 and 2 together, realizing how much your emotions are connected to your eating behaviours.

Sure, we *know* we shouldn't stuff our faces with extra buttery mashed potatoes at dinner, but with the kids fighting at the table and the day you've had, *who cares?!*

And you're not exactly famished when you're back in the kitchen 2 hours later grazing on crackers, chips or anything salty, but you're bored! You've got cravings to indulge, damn it.

Maybe your go-to foods aren't salty, they're sweet and sugary. A couple of Mountain Dews and a pack of M&M's

before that big meeting with the boss, why not? After all, experts say chocolate's good for you!

(Dark chocolate, not those cute little M&M's, *do* have some health benefits. But it's still not broccoli.)

In the face of daily stressors, it feels like willpower is about as real as the boogeyman.

This might seem counterintuitive -- but attempting to exercise willpower is actually one of the WORST things you can do if you're hearings those cravings call out to you.

If relying on willpower is one side of the coin, guilt-ridden emotional eating is the other.

Not a good place to be. The fact is, both the symptoms AND causes of emotional eating are identical to a little word most of us would rather not think about:

Addiction.

It's a topic no one wants to talk about but almost everyone has been touched by.

With a full-on opioid addiction crisis wreaking havoc on families all across North America, I realize that this is a touchy subject, especially for people who've been affected by drug abuse personally. I get it because I've been touched by addiction too.

You may have been raised in a family with alcoholism, drug abuse or other addictions like shopping, hoarding, sex or a workaholic parent. You might currently be in a relationship with someone suffering, like a friend or partner.

Make no mistake about it -- chronic dieting is an addiction like any of those.

Again, I'm not here for finger-wagging; I'm all about soul-empowering. By understanding the hormonal process underlying addiction, so many lightbulbs will go off in your head, your brain might feel like it's imploding.

It's not your fault, you just didn't know what you didn't know. . .until now.

Freedom from emotional eating starts with understanding the feelings associated with food -- and it ends with making peace with your emotions. All of them. Not just the ones you like to hang out with.

Who wouldn't choose joy over anxiety and guilt, right? That's why this chapter and the next few to follow aren't specifically focused on what you should be eating. We'll find our way there in Chapter 9.

For now, I want you to start embracing how you feel without filtering a single emotion. This is the answer to making peace with yourself and your body, and it's what I refer to as Full Frontal Living™.

This chapter kicks off an overview of all the emotional pieces that go into creating lasting change and lasting weight loss, which is what you're after. I want you to stop fighting your emotions and instead work WITH them to create the life you desire.

But it WILL take work on your part. Approaching the science of diet addiction -- like any other addiction -- means our job is to place the burden of change squarely on our own 2 shoulders. I love this quote so much, I turned it into a poster to hang on my wall, "No one is coming to save you. This life is 100% your responsibility."

How's that other saying go? *Point a finger at someone, and three are pointing right back at you.*

It's so easy to point fingers, place blame elsewhere and believe that if your circumstances changed, you'd finally achieve the body and health you want.

You might not like reading this, but taking radical responsibility for your life means no longer being a victim to yourself or other people, places and things.

I didn't write this book to coddle you through the process of change; I'm here to be a truth teller and loving disrupter in your life.

This is messy work, absolutely. But it's worth it. The only way to feel empowered and stay that way for the rest of your life is to look to yourself.

Seriously. Ask yourself, "What's going on in my own life when I want to blame someone else? How am I showing up for myself? What do I need to change from the inside out?"

Things don't change; people change. And if nothing changes, nothing changes. End. Of. Story.

I've witnessed the struggle to create lasting change firsthand -- in my own family. Trust me, when I write about addiction, I know what I'm talking about -- too well.

The way I coach my clients changed forever the moment my husband walked through the doors of an addiction treatment centre seeking help.

Left alone with a 6 month-old baby and 2 young sons, I felt like my world had been ripped out from underneath me. For over a decade, I'd been teaching women how to exercise and change their eating habits so they could lose weight and feel amazing in their bodies.

I started my career as a personal fitness coach, then moved to nutrition when I realized that the physical transformations my clients wanted truly started in the kitchen. That is where my true passion lied, and I set out with the intention to educate as many women as possible around nutrition and body composition change.

I built programs like the ones you're learning about in this book. I was on top of the world until my husband's silent struggle with addiction suddenly spilled out for the world to see.

Truth be told, I kept it a secret. I was TERRIFIED my clients would find out. Only my closest friends and family knew what was happening. I hadn't seen the signs of my husband's struggle even though they were right under my nose!

So suddenly, just like that. . .he was gone. Hubby checked into a 5-month rehab program.

I, determined to "fix" everything, then signed up for group counseling sessions.

I was there to learn how to help my husband and put our lives back together.

Imagine my shock when I realized those counseling sessions had nothing to do with *him*. They were all about *me*.

My stuff.

My stories.

His healing journey became the catalyst for my own transformation when I faced a jolting realization: I was just as sick as he was.

Codependent and addicted to dysfunctional behaviours, unhealthy relationships and in serious denial.

In my own way, I was an addict, too.

I felt crushed, broken and weak.

As I worked through those sessions, I was shocked by what behaviors I uncovered.

I spent my time caretaking everyone, from my hubby to my clients.

I was a total people-pleaser, always overextending myself to make others happy.

I ran from conflict and never said what I meant; keeping the peace was more important than speaking my mind.

I set the bar high and achieved a ton, but I never allowed myself to feel successful.

I hid behind perfectionism so no one could see how insecure I felt.

To move forward, I had to get out of my head and drop into my heart.

I had to feel the emotions I covered with my behaviors.

I had to stop acting like a victim so I could take responsibility for my life and the person I wanted to become.

Although an incredibly painful journey for me, this process turned into the greatest catalyst in my life to push me back to who I really am -- and to embrace ALL parts of me.

And in a twist of irony, watching my husband receive treatment and his personalized plan to stay clean showed me a gaping hole inside the previous edition of the E.A.T! Framework.

I hadn't said a word about the CAUSE of emotional eating.

THAT is the key to freedom from cravings -- and feeling like a slave to the whims of willpower.

Over time, understanding the role self-empowerment plays in overcoming self-destructive, emotion-numbing behaviours showed me how to teach my clients to create their own nutritional blueprints, so they could put their hands back on the wheel of their own health.

Unfortunately, my first hand education also included watching men and women succumb to their addictions after release. I've witnessed relapses, near-deadly overdoses and multiple *repeat* visits to rehab.

In and out of the treatment centre -- it's like yo-yo dieting.

While my hubby was in there, I grieved with families who lost loved ones to addiction. I still cry when I read about anyone losing their battle with addiction.

Make no mistake, addiction of any kind devastates and destroys -- yet it also offers the possibility of personal transformation and a life of wonder you can hardly imagine.

Addiction is a disease, yes; but that doesn't mean we do not wield the dual powers of choice and change.

Addiction does not make you a victim nor does it make you helpless -- far from it.

This was an uncomfortable truth to realize, but that doesn't make it any less true.

In most cases, the women I work with are not struggling with severe food addictions like bulimia, anorexia or morbid obesity. (If you are, PLEASE seek professional help through a local addiction counseling service. Although the tools in the book can help, you must seek deeper healing with the support of counselors and psychologists who are specifically trained in this field.)

My clients don't face death because of their relationship with food, but they do exhibit addictive behaviour patterns driven by the same hormones.

Because of that, they face potentially serious illness and disease -- if they continue to treat their bodies like garbage cans.

As I've already said, food is not a relationship you can avoid or abstain from, but you DO have the power to take back control and maintain healthy boundaries.

However, it's the invisible addiction to dieting (not food) that you can forever put to rest. You might not be able to abstain from eating, but you CAN abstain from diet culture.

With that in mind, I've had to develop a "recovery plan" for people wrestling with food-related addiction -- even if it's under the guise of emotional eating. Let's just tell it like it is, shall we?

Now, in my coaching work, I see women doing the same thing -- but with food.

We've got to stop hiding from our emotions and start acknowledging that they're in the room with us.

So you'd better figure out what works for you; otherwise, you'll be in and out of the nutrition treatment centres known as "diets" for the rest of your life. Believe me, that's no fun.

To put it simply, our emotions can be a prison or a lighthouse. (We both prefer that they be the latter.)

Pay attention to your emotions. Let them be a guiding light to help show you the way, and you'll overcome emotional eating for the rest of your life.

So, why the detour into addiction, drugs and treatment centres?

Because I truly believe that when we know WHY we're driven to eat, that knowledge becomes potential power; we can finally change the cycle of negative behaviour.

Yes, I want you to pay attention to your emotions, but I also want to give you the science behind addiction-driven eating so you realize, *"Wow, I guess I'm normal. There's nothing wrong with me."*

I want everybody to feel normal. Remember, it's *not* about the food! Yes, what you eat is incredibly important, but how you *think* and *feel* about food and your body is really what drives emotional eating.

If we don't do the emotional work to start feeling good enough, accepting ourselves as worthy and loving our bodies as we are now, it will be impossible to leave the treatment centre of dieting for good.

You don't have to like something to accept it, but constantly focusing on and believing that there's something wrong with you or your body will prevent you from thriving.

Thriving isn't something reserved for later. It's available to you NOW.

Like I said, this goes beyond food. Take money, for instance. How many times have you heard the story where somebody comes into a lot of money, only to end up broke again?

You can drop 60 pounds, but if you don't learn to love and accept your body as it is now, you're not going to love it when it's 60 pounds lighter.

My friend and client Keri-Anne described to me what it's like to have the mindset shift so the focus isn't on food, it's on *feelings*.

"Instead of beating myself up about certain behaviours, you reframed it with proof that sometimes our thoughts can trigger a total food addiction moment where we really are powerless to the biology we create with thoughts around food. The trick is to learn how we get triggered and to make different choices before we repeat the cycle."

Proof.

When you know the truth, the truth sets you free.

So, what is the truth about the "total food addiction moments" Keri-Anne describes that we can all relate to?

To put it simply, addiction is a long and powerful influence on the brain that manifests in three ways -- cravings, control and consequences. (This is true for addiction to both cocaine and Coca-Cola.)

You've got cravings. You feel out of control. You know you won't like the consequences, but in the moment they feel like they're worth it.

How many times have you scarfed down that one cookie, and the voice in your head scolds you, "Don't eat 4 more! Your pants won't fit. You'll feel like crap."

Then what happens?

Three more cookies end up in your mouth! Soon after, you beat yourself up.

"Why did I do that? What the hell is wrong with me?"

We all have powerful neurotransmitters that shape behaviours like this. The first one is called dopamine. This is our motivator, this creates the chase.

Dopamine drives us towards pleasure. I'm sure you can remember a time when you first fell in love and wanted to be with that person all the time.

Dopamine never let's "enough be enough," so cravings feel insatiable. It will cause a rat to bore a hole in the wall with their tiny teeth to get to a Fruit Loop on the other side. Dopamine loooooooves sugar, salt and fat in case you hadn't figured that out yet.

It kicks in when you think about your favorite comfort food or see a commercial for it on TV, all of a sudden you have a huge craving that you just can't satisfy until you hop in the car and go get it. There's a reason snacks are always positioned at the checkout counter. Food manufacturers are trying to trigger your dopamine response so you'll buy.

That's all dopamine. The nano-second it starts flowing, the willpower fight is over. Overwhelming cravings take over.

The second hormone that drives our behaviour around feelings and food is called serotonin. This is your pleasure, reward and "feel good" hormone.

In North American culture, from the time we're toddlers, we are programmed to see food as a reward and a comfort. It's used to celebrate the good, bad and the face-down moments in our lives. It brings us together, and it's how we show love.

Food is the common thread that connects us. It's an important part of our cultures and traditions. But we've lost its sacred importance and perspective on the role it *should* play.

How many times have you said to your own kids, "If you just behave for twenty more minutes, then I'll give you a treat," or "If you cooperate with mommy, I'll give you this"?

And when your kids' sports team wins a game, you all go out to celebrate with a pizza or a Slurpee afterwards. Food is used to celebrate and reward ourselves.

We also use food to soothe our aches and pains, and we offer it to others to ease our own discomfort caused by their suffering.

We feed others to make us feel better.

Over time, it's inevitable that unhealthy food becomes attached to feeling good -- higher levels of serotonin released throughout the body. Food becomes a crutch, and a shortcut, to feel better.

A study conducted at Victoria University in Wellington, Australia demonstrated that people who have more addictive tendencies actually have lower levels of serotonin in their bodies. That's why they have stronger cravings for the object of their addiction than others do -- gotta get that serotonin flowin'!

This is similar to people with diabetes, who have to take insulin shots because their body doesn't produce enough of it naturally.

Whether low serotonin levels affect you or not, there are many ways to boost your serotonin in healthy, constructive ways. Getting outside and going for a walk is one. It's simple, and it works.

Regular exercise is also a mood-booster, as is connecting with people you love. I'm passionate about self-care because you raise your serotonin levels by nurturing yourself without turning to food.

The third hormone to be aware of is called oxytocin, otherwise known as the cuddle chemical. This is released when you're engaging in a loving way with your kids, when you're giving someone a hug or after enjoying intimacy with your partner.

When we get a rush of oxytocin, we feel the most connected to ourselves and to other people. It's well noted for it's appearance in breastfeeding mamas.

Without that connection to ourselves or others, addiction THRIVES. Check out Johann Hari's *New York Times* bestselling book *Chasing the Scream* and his TED Talk *Everything you think you know about addiction is wrong.*

Johann makes the point that addiction is caused less by chemical "hooks" and more by a lack of human connection.

I do want you to be aware of chemical hooks like dopamine, but know that *connection* matters more in your fight to make peace with food and your body. That's why we use food to move away from emotions we don't like -- we're not feeling connected with ourselves, and we're not acknowledging the way we're feeling.

That's why people in the addiction recovery community sit down and connect with each other bedhind closed doors, sharing stories and feeling seen and heard. They enjoy the benefits of dopamine, serotonin and oxytocin in a healthy, intimate environment. Their needs are fulfilled without the object of addiction, and they finally begin to heal.

So when those cravings hit and the hormones flow, you DO have the ability to skip straight to what your body needs. All habits and behaviours can be changed IF you're willing to start getting conscious about what's happening and tune into what your body actually needs. And hey, sometimes a craving is just a craving. Who doesn't occasionally want a sweet or salty treat?

But when your cravings are a daily struggle and take over your life, you feel out of control. Yet you continue to engage in the behaviour knowing the consequences. THAT is when you know you're up against more than just the average cookie craving!

In that moment, you have a choice to take a different action. To give yourself the connection you need to sidestep your cravings.

You CAN do things that get serotonin and oxytocin flowing to break the cycle of cravings. The simple act of reaching out and connecting with a friend -- instead of reaching for that carton of Ben & Jerry's or body-checking your kid for his lollipop -- will kibosh your cravings. At the very least, you'll give yourself a fighting chance.

When you do sense that struggle coming on, pay attention to those feelings. Laugh at yourself! I am completely serious. Don't make food into this epic deal where you act like you've personally failed if you eat something that isn't going to support your weight loss.

Reaching out to connect doesn't make you weak. In fact, its impact is the exact opposite. You'll find a strength you never knew you had.

Keep the question, "What do I need?" tucked in your back pocket when a friend isn't available. That way, you can fulfill your body's request for dopamine, serotonin or oxytocin in a healthy way.

Now that we've worked our way through the science of addiction, I want to reiterate that not everyone is a food addict in the clinical sense. There absolutely ARE folks who have been in and out of recovery from not just drug and alcohol addiction relapses, but food as well. Bulimia, anorexia, obesity and life-threatening overeating are all addictions.

At the same time, not everybody is going to be at that severe end of the spectrum. Having an extra drink doesn't make you an alcoholic, for instance. Neither does chowing down on an extra slice of whipped cream-topped pie. Only you know where you fall on the spectrum.

I hope this book helps you see things with a new perspective and gives you some insight into your struggles. Remember how I wrote earlier that the truth will set you free?

Well, it will first piss you off! If you're feeling a little flustered after reading how our triple hormonal threat can drive addiction to food. . .*good*.

You may want to exercise your willpower just to prove me wrong, but that's literally the exact opposite of what I recommend to my clients who want BIG TIME results.

When the dopamine starts flowing, relying on your own grit and determination to keep your hands off that candy bar will get you nowhere.

With so many demands in our daily lives, we exhaust it quickly. It's renewable, but we burn through it quickly. Just getting out of bed in the morning without hitting the snooze button 3 or 4 times drains it.

Thinking it will be available by the time that the buffet dinner rolls around is unreasonable. So stop beating yourself up for not having enough of it.

That's why you need to be aware of each emotion's presence the moment you feel it, and choose instead to adjust your patterns with a spirit of compassion and empathy.

Changing patterns when the cravings are screaming takes both time and tenacity, but the key is to *feel your feelings filter-free* -- now that's a tongue-twister -- and step into Full Frontal Living™.

Instead of obeying those cravings, sit back for a moment to just "be" with your emotions. Pay attention to the feeling beneath the craving, and acknowledge why it's there.

Did you get in a fight with your boss? Poor night's sleep? Kids driving you up (and down) the walls?

Stop trying to avoid what you're feeling by feeding it.

As you do this -- and I'll show you exactly how before closing out this chapter -- you will start to feel like my client Saleema, who shared with me, " I am no longer afraid of food. My body is changing shape and I feel revived!"

SO many good things happen when you stop playing the willpower game.

Break that cycle, and just listen to your body. You're not broken, and there's nothing you need to fix. The emotional eating you've struggled with has simply masked deeper, unmet needs.

So let's identify those needs, start to meet them and set your emotions free.

Honestly, when was the last time you asked yourself how you were feeling? I mean actually *asked* yourself personally, even out loud.

It's a scary question. When life isn't all peaches and cream, we really don't want to know the answer. We don't want to face the darker emotions of anger, resentment or fear.

Whenever those emotions start to exert control over our mood, we say to ourselves in an accusatory tone, "Why am I feeling this way? I don't want to feel like this. I don't want to feel upset. I don't want to cry. I don't want to be anxious."

We make it *wrong* to feel what we're feeling instead of just allowing ourselves to be curious. We second-guess the message our feelings tell us, and we do our damndest to run away from them.

Just how lopsided is that though? We never, ever interrogate ourselves when we wake up feeling happy, joyful or excited. If we don't question or judge enthusiasm, then why are we questioning and judging anger or anxiety?

Emotions are neither good nor bad; they're simply colors on a rainbow. As a human being, you get a full spectrum. Any rainbow that tries to hide its purple or its blue is concealing its true nature. Imagine if a rainbow was just one stripe of colour; it wouldn't be nearly as spectacular.

When you run away from "bad" emotions, you never let yourself be truly, truly sad -- or truly, truly happy. Life becomes a constant battle to hold the emotional territory labeled, "Okay," or my personal favourite, "Fine."

The truth is, we feel most alive when we are extremely joyful and when we sink to the depths of sadness. I don't know about you, but when I've lost somebody that I really loved, it's a full body emotional experience. It is SO painful, I know I am alive. No, it doesn't feel good. Grief totally sucks, but that's how emotions work. Light needs darkness for us to appreciate both.

Feelings won't kill us, so why do we fight them? The more we push back, the more they hold us hostage.

Emotions are energy, they want to move. So instead of judging them, get curious and allow them to be there. Feel what's there for you. Then, let them move through you.

To keep this new response pattern handy, I want you to keep in mind 2 acronyms.

The first is **P. A. I. N.** -- Pay Attention Inward Now. Whenever your feelings pull you towards a numbing behaviour that you know isn't aligned with your ideal health, gently check in with yourself.

"How am I feeling? How am I feeling?"

Your body will tell you what it *really* needs when you ask it.

The second acronym that will empower you to recognize your triggers and make different choices is **H. A. L. T.** -- Hungry, Angry/Anxious, Lonely, Tired.

Whenever you experience two or more H. A. L. T. triggers at the same time, exercising willpower is like using a paper bag as a shield to stop a cannonball.

Instead, avoid these triggers altogether by allowing yourself to feel them unfiltered.

As you're doing that, take radical responsibility to support yourself. This is Full Frontal Living™ unfolding! As a result, you're going to find your freedom and take back control.

If you go hours without eating, hunger will end up sending you face-down into a bag of Doritos. So whenever you feel a rumbly in the tumbly, ask yourself, "When was the last time I ate?"

Then *immediately* make a healthy choice. Stop whatever you're doing, and listen to your body before it's too late.

When you feel angry or anxious, give yourself permission to let that energy flow on through while you're just hanging out with it. If you don't, you'll be reaching for a way to numb it. If you haven't eaten for hours, your ability to resist something sweet or salty is a pipe dream at best.

I guarantee that when you don't try to shove your emotions away like a toddler having a tantrum, they'll run their course, and you'll be able to go on your merry way.

Seriously though, what's the best way to calm a four year-old's tantrum? Let them freak out, and 10 minutes later, they'll be over it. They won't even remember what triggered the madness in the first place!

So as you're going through the day, "H. A. L. T." when a craving points you in the direction of a snack that doesn't support your weight loss. Stay grounded for a few minutes and allow yourself to think.

"Wait a minute. What's going on for me right now? Am I really hungry, or am I just tired and really pissed off that my husband said that thing?"

We're not used to responding this way to stress, are we? Normally, we'd just put our head down and hope willpower can deliver.

It usually doesn't though, does it?

The next step is to KNOW the pieces of H.A.L.T. that trigger you *before* they show up.

I seriously do not screw with my sleep because I know that if I don't get enough rest, my cravings are going to be off the hook. Pair that with not having healthy food on the regular, and I might as well drive directly to the corner store for a bag of sour gummies.

This is how you take your power back and be radically responsible for how you want to feel, what you want to achieve. Don't put yourself in the position of feeling powerless.

Because you aren't.

When I first taught the P.A.I.N. and H.A.L.T. responses to students in my signature *Feelings & Food* program, people resisted. Years and years of defaulting to willpower can keep people locked in a prison of inaction.

So as you pay attention to your emotions, know that resistance does not make you abnormal. Just breathe.

And get curious. Your resistance isn't there to piss you off, but to show you the way. It's linked to fear and to the discomfort of not following the usual path.

A wise coach once said to me, "Your comfort zone isn't really comfortable, it's just familiar."

Resistance shows up when we try to break away from what's familiar. It's just part of being human. So instead of fighting it, call out what you're afraid of by name.

Are you afraid my method of feeling your feelings won't work -- or that it will?

Are you afraid of how you'll feel when you don't self-censor those emotions? If so, what's the worst thing that's going to happen?

What would you be giving up if you changed these patterns? What beliefs would you have to let go of, and what would that mean?

Think about it. *What do you believe you'd have to give up if you no longer obsessed about your weight?*

We use dieting to give ourselves permission to eat what we want, when we want it, because unconsciously we KNOW we'll just be going on a diet anyways.

The resistance you feel is your brain literally trying to keep you happy, comfortable and safe. It's like a well-meaning friend who gives you unwanted advice on the regular. Your brain "thinks" it knows what you want and need based on past behaviours.

Again, this is human nature. I'm certainly not immune. That same struggle has carried over into my business.

For years, I hid in plain sight. I felt terrified of networking and meeting new people. The thought of having to introduce myself and talk about who I was and how I helped people made me want to turtle in bed under my duvet.

You can imagine how this would make growing a successful business nothing short of a miracle. Truth be told, networking wasn't the problem. I was simply afraid of being judged! Of not feeling good enough, smart enough or successful enough. I was terrified of what "they" would think.

After getting down to the nitty-gritty, I documented those fears in my journal. The simple act of naming my fears made me realize, "Wow, none of these are really that bad."

That exercise also made me realize that if I was going to show up in a bigger way in my business, I would have to stop judging myself every step of the way.

On the flip side, I also looked at the best possible outcome of attending an event. I imagined meeting a few amazing people who I'd have a really deep connection with, who could turn into friends, collaborators or clients. I also acknowledged that no matter what happened, whether I was judged by someone or not. . .*life would go on*.

The truth is, I'd never know if anyone judged me. As a rule of thumb, it's important to know that how others think and feel about you is NONE of your business anyways.

Let that wisdom nugget land for a second; you'll have the chance to do something with it at the end of this chapter.

But before we get there, we have to take a look at something else first -- we cannot find freedom in the present if we're still chained to the past. Not going to happen.

Those stories of the past, even if you've forgotten them, play on repeat inside our subconscious. That's why so many women find pattern change to be an impossible task. They don't know how they developed the patterns they have now in the first place -- or why!

Engage in some introspective self-care with me. How have you felt about yourself up until this point in your life?

How do you want to feel about yourself going forward? Have you always wanted to feel that way?

What has been your relationship with food and your body in the past?

What is your family history around addiction? What did you grow up with?

To release your past means that you actually look at it -- without judgement, guilt or shame. Just a dash of curiosity.

Do you have a family history of addiction? Maybe it's not your mother or father but an uncle, an aunt or a grandfather. Maybe it was drugs or alcohol. Maybe you had a cousin who exercised like a crazy fiend. Maybe you lived with a hoarder or someone who shopped 'til they dropped, but every sentence out of their mouth was a complaint about money and debt.

Do you recognize any of these patterns within yourself?

On one side of my own family, there was alcoholism. With alcoholism came codependent behaviours of people living with the addict. Caretaking, control, perfectionism, people-pleasing, constant worrying, covering up for other people's crap, being passive aggressive and living life with little attention paid to putting your own needs first. Each of these behaviours mesh with addiction.

Even if you aren't an addict to food per se, codependent behaviours are just as much of an addiction. They can take over your life and will be the fuel for emotional eating -- and all other forms of substance abuse.

Brené Brown put it this way, "Codependency is to addiction as salt water is to a man dying of thirst."

If you give a thirsty man salt water, he will die.

Codependency and addiction are so intertwined, it's hard to know which came first. They simply perpetuate the existence of each other!

Codependent behaviours keep us feeling small in our lives so we don't actually live for ourselves. We feel like we're suffocating, like there's no room to ever make a change.

Before my friend and client Jennifer saw the pounds and inches start to disappear, she had to do the inner work of reflection -- and actually feel her own feelings.

"I was overweight my entire life. I had no idea what it felt like to be healthy, to have energy, to not be ashamed of my body. You carry that with you and people feel it."

I'm so happy for Jennifer -- she fundamentally changed the relationship she has with her body because she acknowledged the stories from the past that held her back.

That's why looking at your past and paying attention is SO empowering.

The truth will set you free, but it will first piss you off.

Are you pissed off yet?

PROGRESS, NOT PERFECTION

You will face resistance as you create a new normal and step outside of what's familiar. Remember, you are not powerless. Dig into the questions below to prepare your mind -- and your emotions -- for the times you would have otherwise reached for junk food. Create healthy patterns, get healthy results.

Name your fear and resistance.

What's the best thing that could happen?

What's the worst thing that could happen?

What will probably happen?

Repeat this exercise every time you experience resistance. Remember, ALWAYS LEAD WITH CURIOSITY.

Chapter 3
Falling in Love with You

"Because I said so."

When I was a kid, I heard adults say this to me repeatedly. In fact, I probably heard it hundreds of times between my parents, teachers and family friends.

Granted, I wasn't the most agreeable kid, constantly challenging authority and questioning everything. It could be argued that I deserved this response because no answer would have satisfied me unless I got my way!

Why can't I go to the mall on Sunday?

Why do I need to wait 'til after class to ask for help?

Why do I need to be home by nine?

Why do I need to know my multiplication tables?

Why, why, why, why?

None of the answers made any sense to me. Take math, for example. I hated it, and it hated me. I knew Accounting would never make the short list of viable career paths.

Since the teacher was there to teach us during school hours, why did I have to wait until after the bell rang to get extra help?

Now that I'm a parent, I get it. Kids ask a LOT of questions!

But I realize now that I wasn't challenging authority, I was simply exercising extreme curiosity and learning to think outside the box. Even at a young age, I knew the status quo didn't serve me.

Unfortunately, what parents, teachers and friends used to just shut me up turned into fuel for a lifelong battle with insecurity. Since I was a kind, I'd had this nagging feeling that I was wrong or stupid, and that I didn't have anything of value to contribute to a conversation.

You have nothing important to say. Nobody wants to hear you. You don't know what you're talking about.

To my young ears, "Because I said so," meant my opinion had no value. I should learn to just keep my mouth shut.

Of course, no loving mother or father wants their child to enter adulthood believing these useless ideas -- especially since they were entirely untrue.

But that's exactly what happened.

The subconscious beliefs I anchored in at an early age about not being good enough, smart enough or worthy enough shaped the years ahead, creating serious problems as my career began.

Even though I'm passionate about what I do, I've had to exercise my "courage" muscle every day my feet have hit the floor. All because my internal default had me believe my opinion was about as valuable as the dust inside a vacuum cleaner. It's taken me years to get comfortable with public speaking, being visible, being a leader, realizing I'm smart and knowing that what I have to say is incredibly valuable. Writing and publishing a book was never on my radar until recently because of these reasons.

We all have beliefs born out of stories. Although the symptoms might vary, at our core, we're all up against the same thing -- The human need to feel love, safe and *to belong*.

In the previous chapter, we got to the root of emotional eating triggers, why they're totally natural and how we can use our emotions as a lighthouse to point the way to healthier behaviors.

Now, let's dig even deeper. I'm talking more than just feelings. Let's talk about the stories that bring them up.

Maybe Auntie Helen told you that you'd be perfect if you lost five pounds. Maybe somebody told you that you were built like a boy. Maybe your teacher told you that you were the smart one in the class, or not the pretty one.

In my case, when I was a teenager, some kid yelled out his pickup truck window, "Nice forehead!"

I assumed his comment was directed at me, so I took it to mean that my forehead was grotesquely large. From that moment on, I never had a hairstyle without bangs -- or "fringe," as my Aussie friends call it.

That experience was a defining moment for me. I let someone else's (bad) opinion become my truth and, in the process, handed away my power. Words became a story I believed with all my heart.

Not only was I convinced I had the biggest forehead on the planet, I also believed that *someone else* could have an opinion (that mattered) about MY body.

Nothing could be further from the truth. But I hear similar stories time and time again from my clients. I still remember Lea, who confessed during our first session that her downward spiral into eating disorders began the moment her then-boyfriend told her she'd be perfect. . .if only she dropped 10 pounds.

This young woman was, and still is, one of the most beautiful people I know -- inside and out. But she, too, fell prey to the belief that *someone else's opinion about her body mattered more than her own.*

A couple of years ago, my oldest son asked me, "Mom, how come you never pull your hair back in a tight ponytail?"

I caught myself about to say, "Because I have a huge forehead."

Those words on the tip of my tongue made me laugh. All of a sudden, the truth clicked. That statement felt absurd coming out of my own mouth! Yet I'd let that belief live inside my brain -- planted by some random dude I didn't even know -- guide my behavior (and hairstyles) for more than 20 years.

Whether or not my forehead is large is irrelevant. Only *I* get to decide how I think and feel about my body.

So, I pulled back my hair into a ponytail. Yes, it felt weird the first few times. Vulnerable. Exposed. That was a part of me that I'd learned to hide. But the fact was, I had no reason to hide it in the first place. It's big, bold and beautiful. And it's all mine. Seriously, I'm not sure how I lived without my go-to 5-days-a-week hairstyle!

The truth is, we all come into this world perfect -- exactly the way we're supposed to be. But whether it's well-meaning parents or some bratty boy in a truck, not far out of the gate we pick up different ideas.

We're not good enough. If only we were different. If only we changed certain things, that would make us okay.

Consider the stories in your own life. Imagine how many of them are feeding you a bunch of BS you didn't even know you're carting around.

What nasty little nuggets have you picked up from somebody else?

In this chapter, you're going to uncover the moments in your life that defined your relationship with your body and with food. You'll take a closer look at whether or not these stories are serving you today and, if not, how to strip them off your soul.

We're only able to accept our bodies -- and love our bodies -- when we realize that no one but WE have the privilege of deciding how we think and feel about ourselves.

My friend Tara gets it. Even though she hasn't reached her own ideal point in her weight loss journey, she loves herself. She accepts herself. No except's, but's or if only's.

After a live session working through the E.A.T! Framework, Tara told me, "I am learning to love me. I am able to look in the mirror and love myself. I love all my curves!"

Go, Tara, go!

She's purged the negative stories about her body and her health from her life because they don't serve her anymore. In fact, they never did.

Think of this emotional and mental purging like it's a closet. You've got to get rid of all those old clothes you're never going to wear. You held onto that smaller size, hoping you'd get there someday. What if that piece of clothing is what's holding you back? It's a constant reminder of the times you felt like you failed in the past. It's tormenting you! Just give the damn thing away.

The same goes for clothes in your wardrobe that are a larger size. By keeping them in your closet, you tell yourself that there is no way you can keep the weight off that you've worked so hard to lose.

Purge. That. Shit.

Stepping into the future you want for yourself means releasing the one you don't.

There's nothing righteous about punishing ourselves. Think about it; if you're a parent, do you ignore your child every single day? Do you tell your child how much you hate him? Do you tell her she's not good enough, that she's a horrible little nobody? Do you remind him that he's worthless? Do you withhold love and affection until she's more "deserving"?

Of course not! You'd have a miserable human being on your hands who couldn't cope in society. She'd constantly misbehave and act out. Any child who feels like she isn't loved or isn't good enough is a very unhappy one.

So, why do we talk to ourselves that way? Why do we allow stories to play on repeat inside our heads? They just melt our confidence like an ice cube on a sidewalk in August.

I want you to think about how you talk to yourself every day, especially when it comes to your body. This reveals how much you love yourself.

Your body is not separate from you. **Your body is you**. Pay attention to the shit you say to it day in and day out about how you don't like this, how that isn't good enough.

Why do I have to look and feel so crappy? Why can't I weigh less? Why can't I lose this stupid muffin top?

You're disgusted with yourself for no good reason. Even if you THINK you're justified in believing all that shit, I'm telling you, you are NOT. You're creating a toxic environment for your body, and that's not okay.

Think about it. It's not okay for you to talk like that to your kids. It's not okay for you to talk like that to your friends.

And it's certainly not okay for you to talk like that to yourself.

If you want a body that looks and feels amazing ·· which is the whole point of the E.A.T! Framework ·· you absolutely will not get there unless you start to learn to love yourself. And that starts with how you think and feel about your body.

Give yourself love. Because if you keep condemning your body, it's never going to show up and love you back, ever.

Call me a ranty pants if you'd like, but I've seen thousands of women like Tara finally see the results they've dreamed of only *after* they chose to love themselves -- no matter what.

So, what needs to change for you?

First off, make it no longer okay to say to yourself what you wouldn't say to your own child or you best friend. Stop working against yourself.

Then, appreciate the fact that your body is doing its absolute best to be your faithful servant, and your faithful companion.

It keeps you ALIVE, so in return, how about you show it some gratitude? If falling in love with your body feels like too much of a stretch, at least attempt to start *liking* it more. You don't have to like everything about it to fall in love with it.

Your body wants you to *move*. It wants you to *run*. It wants you to *play*. It wants you to *feel amazing*.

Your body just wants you to be happy. If you put junk beliefs or junk food in it, how is that loving to yourself?

Seriously, who wants to get up every day and not like themselves starting from the moment the alarm clock goes off? That's no way to live. We can do better.

My client Lou put a simple but powerful reminder up on her mirror.

"BE KIND."

This prompt slowly changed how she felt about her body. It helped her keep those toxic thoughts in check. She committed to no longer making it okay to talk smack about her appearance.

Now, Lou enjoys a peaceful relationship with her body that makes eating to nurture it a no-brainer.

Imagine if you wrote a love letter to yourself in 2nd person, if you addressed yourself as the total and complete person that you are.

Your note could be as short as Lou's or as long as a sonnet by Shakespeare. The truth is, you're pretty damn spectacular.

When writing your love letter, you'd have every reason to acknowledge yourself. To brag. To shine. To be seen *and* heard.

I don't care if you were told that loving yourself was unnatural, egotistical or selfish. They were wrong. Learning to receive praise from others -- and yourself -- is critical to cultivating a greater sense of self worth, self love and feelings of enoughness.

Giving myself nightly high-fives is part of my daily self care routine. It has nothing to do with ego. It's just a way of reminding myself how awesome I am.

YOU are awesome, too. If you're alive and kicking, you're awesome for just having made it this far. Given that you're reading this book, I do, in fact, assume you're alive!

You deserve to be celebrated. Just because you were given stories that made you believe otherwise doesn't make any of them true.

I now make a conscious effort to compliment and uncomfortable myself out loud. Literally, I pat myself on the back and say, "Wow, look how capable you are at this! Lisa, you're a freakin' ROCK STAR!"

If this kind of self-praise feels completely fake and uncomfortable when you try it for yourself, that means the false belief-riddled stories you've told yourself have GOT to go. Remember what I said about discomfort in Chapter 2? *It shows up to show us the way.* If I'm stirring up some strong emotions, GREAT! That means I've hit on something big, so it's time to blow the lid off the emotional crap you've been carrying around without knowing it.

Let's reframe the defining moments of your relationship with your body so you can feel loved and safe enough to shower yourself with praise that feels genuine.

Reframing simply means to change the way you look at something, which changes the way you feel about it.

For example, I reframed my defining moment of the forehead incident by getting clear on what that story made me believe about my appearance. By asking me a simple question, my son gave me an opportunity to reframe this story. I was finally able to see how ridiculous it was. The result was a new perspective about how I saw my forehead and who gets to have a say about my body. I now wear whatever hairstyle I want without any feelings of shame. That simple reframing moment gave me my power back because I was willing to get curious and question *why* I believed it.

The revolutionary teacher Louise Hay put it best, "Every experience I have is perfect for my growth."

It's all in the way you look at those experiences. Perspective changes everything.

Will they hold you back?

Or will you reframe them so they set you free?

As with anything. . .

It's *your* choice.

PROGRESS NOT PERFECTION

What do you believe about your body? What do you believe about dieting? What do you believe about healthy food? What do you believe about losing weight and keeping it off?

Each of those beliefs came from a story. Many times, these stories are based on something misguided that someone else told us, or even on something we innocently picked up along life's way.

In this exercise, reframe each of those stories. Move into your past back to those "moments" when your beliefs first got "defined."

When you write these stories down, you're defanging the beast. Their power is gone, and you're on your way to being FREE of them.

In the space provided below, first, list out your beliefs using the prompts above. List everything you can think of.

Defining Moment #1

Lesson Learned (How Does This Event Serve You?)

Defining Moment #2

Lesson Learned (How Does This Event Serve You?)

Defining Moment #3

Lesson Learned (How Does This Event Serve You?)

Now consider this. . .

What does hanging onto these beliefs allow you to keep doing? Which ones are you ready to release?

Write a breakup letter to your stories expressing how each of these events made you feel. Include what and who you need to forgive (don't forget yourself) and then burn it. It's time to let go of your past so you can step into the future and who you want to become.

Chapter 4
Your Coach, Your Critic, Your Choice

"'Fine is not a feeling, Lisa."

I sat in my very first group therapy session, silenced by the counselor's mic drop moment.

My world had come apart. The word "busy" was my badge of honour and the default setting in life. My mind and emotions were about as organized as a spider web after a hailstorm.

After introducing myself to the other men and women present, all of whom were there to deal with (or so we thought) an addict in the family, the counselor asked each of us how we felt.

"Fine," was my go-to response.

After the counselor challenged that, I realized how out of touch I was. How did I *actually* feel? It's almost like I didn't want to know the answer myself. I was so caught up in my thoughts of how to "fix" the shit storm that my life had become, I had no idea how I actually felt about anything.

Never before had I slowed down, tuned in and listened to what was going on inside my body.

She asked me to get out of my head and drop into my heart. All I could do was glare at her. I'm pretty sure I snapped back, but I only remember her sitting there calmly and silently watching me. I had no idea what she meant, and I saw NO value in feeling my way through the mess. I just needed to find a way out of it. I was PISSED that she wasn't giving me a *How to Fix Addiction* handbook.

Until that meeting, I had denied how I felt. That was the first day I can remember ever letting my anger out and starting to feel my own feelings.

In the silence of the counselor's stare, I couldn't run away. There was nothing in that moment to "do". Behind my anger came a tidal wave of sadness, frustration, confusion and every messy emotion you can imagine.

Something you need to know about me is the fact that I'm tenacious as a grizzly bear hunting for its first meal after hibernation. I never accept the status quo. When I'm determined, not much can stop me.

When another counselor told me that very few relationships survive addiction, I decided to prove him wrong.

But this was the moment I realized, the only relationship that needed to survive was *mine*.

With myself.

From that day in the therapy group forward, I opened myself up to transformation. I chose to become a caring, kind coach for myself. The kind who believes in you, who inspires you to believe in yourself, who pushes you to do your very best.

I decided to give myself the same compassion, empathy and understanding I'd been giving my clients without judgement for my entire career. I opened myself up to vulnerability and dismantled the walls I had built around me.

Through this book, I invite you to do the same.

As we approach the journey that is the E.A.T! framework a few chapters from now, I want you to feel completely prepared for what's to come.

Yes, you'll be creating new habits to replace old ones. Yes, there will be uncomfortable spots. But whether or not you experience the change you desire comes down to your conscious choice to be your own best coach, or your worst critic.

This commitment is simple, as are the wisest choices in life. *Simple*.

To silence the critic and empower the coach, slow down. Pay attention. A healthy relationship between feelings and food will require regular check-ins with yourself. You can't change what you're not conscious of, and *this* is your wake up call.

As you learned in Chapter 2, being with yourself means being with your emotions not trying to move away from them as fast as possible.

When you're feeling super happy, you don't go, "Oh, my goodness, why am I so happy? I need to figure out why I'm so happy. I shouldn't feel so happy, I should watch a tearjerker to pull me out of this happy mood!"

So why then, when you're feeling anxious, angry or frustrated, do you try to escape these emotions?

I get it, they don't feel good. Anxiety is no fun, and I've had depression on my dance card before. But when we do everything in our power to turn these feelings off, they only grow stronger. Emotions are powerful and don't take kindly to being stuffed down. More than that, they don't care much for your judgment.

Imagine a world where we stopped making anxiety, depression, frustration and anger *wrong*! What if we just allowed them to hang out and run their course? I promise, when you commit to doing the inner work and start talking about how you're feeling, they WILL move along. Just like waves rolling in and out on the shore, emotions come and go. And usually. . .just as quickly.

Remember the analogy of the kid with the tantrum? That's powerful energy you're trying to control, and there's a price to be paid when you do. Numbing behaviours like over-eating, over-spending, drinking, doing drugs or just being so fucking busy you don't know if you're coming or going. . .these behaviours destroy your health, your relationships and your sense of connection and belonging.

The very things we want the most are the things we're pushing away, and all because we're unwilling to be with and talk about how we're feeling.

Slow down. Get in touch. Drop into your heart and ask yourself:

"How do I feel today?"

I want you to start your mornings this way. The moment your feet hit the floor, check in with yourself and ask.

Then pay attention, not judging the response. Not making it right or wrong. Just tune into the feeling.

Don't make the same mistake I did. "Good," "Bad" or "Fine" are not feelings.

Let's use the extensive vocabulary we have to call out our feelings by name.

For example, do you feel overwhelmed?

Name that feeling. Just be with it. Curiosity and judgement can't hang out together so when you allow yourself to go deeper you'll get to know yourself more intimately. Why are you feeling overwhelmed? and what are the emotions buried under the overwhelm? Let your body speak freely.

Anxious. . . Confused. . . Insecure. . .

Give your emotions the megaphone of silence.

How else do you feel?

Insignificant. . . Helpless. . . Scared. . .

Soon, what started as just the feeling of overwhelm be-comes a road map to your inner world. Your subconscious beliefs are revealed. No longer do you have to run from an unseen and unknown enemy. We have the power to change when we create conscious awareness and stop making our emotions out to be "wrong" when they feel uncomfortable. Suddenly, the overwhelm reveals the bigger picture of how you're thinking and feeling and what you're running from.

The same goes for other emotions as well -- joy, for example.

Do you feel excited and daring? Creative and playful? Hopeful and optimistic?

When you start to feel your feelings, explore them and get curious, the voice of your inner critic will become crystal clear. You'll start to hear the toxic whispers fuel-ling your anxiety, insecurities and overwhelm. This is the voice that interjects opinions you'd rather not have, likes to consume your thoughts with nothing but negativity and has a way of unravelling your mood if left unchecked.

"You're not good enough, look at your body today. . . You're a horrible mother, you can't keep a clean enough house. . . Why can't you get off your ass and exercise?"

But guess what -- *you* are your critic which means you have the power to shut it down. It's time for your inner coach to step up and say, "You know what? You need to sit down and zip it, critic!"

You've got to stop bullying yourself.

There is a lesson to be learned from some of the great-est coaches in sports. For example, the history-breaking Olympic athlete and track and field coach Bobbie Rosen-feld, and eight-time college basketball coach Pat Summitt *never* used shame to inspire their players to achieve more.

A critic makes a terrible coach. Again, look at sports -- the coaches who lash out at their teams are those that earn terrible reputations and soon find themselves unemployed.

Shame uses the language that enforces the belief "I am bad"and keeps people locked in behaviours that don't serve them. Remember shame fuels addiction and vise versa.

Let's say you eat that triple chocolate chip cookie at the party after you promised yourself no sugar that day.

What does the critic say?

"Wow, I TOTALLY suck! Why don't I have any willpower? I'm never going to get this. I'll never be thin enough. I'll never be light enough. I'll never be pretty enough."

This shaming language does you no good. A coach, on the other hand, offers a very different response as you wipe the last cookie crumbs off your chin. A coach looks for a perspective that provides growth, learning and opportunity. Great coaches are compassionate, caring and encourage us to try again, all while keeping us focused on what we want and why we want it.

"Oh, I ate that. But it's not a big deal. I take responsibility for my choices. What can I reflect on so I can do better next time and not fall prey to my cravings?"

Coaches aren't looking for perfection, just progress. They know success comes from playing the long game and having a growth mindset.

With shame, you never, ever get to be good enough. That's not okay! Instead, I want you to listen to and strengthen your inner coach, who is all about embracing where you're at, accepting your emotions, taking responsibility and changing those patterns.

Coaching thousands of women during my career has shown me why it can be so difficult to change the conversation in your head about your body and your health.

In 2005, the National Science Foundation published research on human thoughts throughout the day day. The average person has between 12,000 and 60,000 thoughts... *per day*.

Of those, 80% are negative. And you want to know the most discouraging part of the study?

A sickening 95% of those negative thoughts are the exact same ones you experienced the day before.

Clearly, one of the biggest things that can hold you back is the way you speak to yourself. Most of us have a constant unkind inner dialogue.

The cure to this self-shaming -- and to breaking free of unhealthy behaviours -- is to stop and listen to your thoughts. Is that inner voice your coach or a critic? Kind or cruel? Is it the voice of shame or guilt? Your best friend or a bullying bitch?

To borrow the sports metaphor again, a coach isn't just there to encourage you. A coach's job is to get you moving in the right direction *toward* something.

That's what diet programs miss when it comes to self-talk. They aren't paying attention to what you're saying to yourself before, during or after your "diet."

They don't look at what beliefs are driving the bus or if those beliefs are supportive or destructive. They want you to just DO your way through weight loss without focusing on who you need to become, the new beliefs you need to anchor in or how to support yourself through the change process.

Harnessing the power of your inner coach will help you *win*, and help you experience the breakthroughs you've always dreamed of.

In Chapter 1, you asked yourself what you wanted -- and whether or not those were really about you. To turn those "wants" into "haves," you need a breakthrough. And every breakthrough I've seen my clients enjoy has had 3 components: the What, the How and the Why.

The What is your dream, the How is your process and the Why is your inspiration.

For example, your What could be, "I want to wear a little black dress." Your How is, "I will make choices about the thoughts I think and the actions I take to support me looking and feeling my best." And the Why is, "I deserve to feel sexy and vibrant."

The best coaches help their players define the dream, keep them on track with the right process and empower them with a purpose that inspires them to be with, and work through resistance.

Be your own best coach. Keep that Why front and center; the How and What will naturally fall into place.

One exercise that I have students in the *Feelings & Food* program complete equips their inner coach to say the right thing at the right time.

When the critic mouths off about that extra helping of lasagna you had in office break room. . .

When you wonder if you'll ever see the number on the scale drop. . .

When you break the number one diet rule of not shopping while hungry. . .

Let your coach remind you who you are.

I AM beautiful. . . I AM deserving. . . I AM enough. . . I AM pretty. . . I AM smart. . . I AM lovable.

Put the emphasis on the "I am" part of the mantra. These simple phrases affirm how you want to feel about yourself. Like an athlete, you are playing to win. So talk to yourself like it!

After a few weeks of consistently coaching themselves, women I work with start to see something miraculous happen. Before, they felt powerless to their cravings, a victim of their own poor choices. But get that coach in there telling it like it is, and the critic starts to lose it's power. Pretty soon, they become their own role models.

The difference between this dramatic change and business as usual is where that drive comes from -- is it external or internal? Are you feeling *motivated* or are you becoming *inspired*?

Motivation looks outside ourselves, and is the belief that if we do more, we'll fix the problem.

It has its time and place, but like willpower, it's short lived at best. It puts our focus on what we don't want, and we use it to try to escape our suffering.

We've got an extra 20 pounds we don't want, so we "get motivated" to run a half marathon and get on a new diet plan someone else came up with.

Motivation always focuses on the negative thoughts, beliefs and feelings you're trying to outrun. It doesn't require you to take responsibility for changing. It's gone as soon as your suffering returns to tolerable levels. It's about as sustainable for creating lasting weight loss as a match is without any fuel to keep the fire burning. It just fizzles out in a puff of smoke.

Sure, we can find examples of people who've initially used motivation to get started, but it was their growing passion for the conditions, activity or circumstance that eventually took over and kept them going.

They ditched motivation, upgraded to inspiration and fundamentally became a new person who embodied the belief of what was possible. Sadly, this rarely happens for those of us trying to lose weight because we get trapped in the addictive cycle of dieting.

There are very few women I know who've actually gotten up one day and decided to run a marathon for the fun of it. They convince themselves that the feeling of the breeze blowing through their hair is going to make them feel fantastic, they just know it.

Most pick up running because they decided they need to lose weight, and running is supposed to be an easy way to help with that. These women aren't waking up inspired to run, they're motivated by something they're not happy with -- the number on the scale or the muffin top peeking over their pants.

Inspiration, on the other hand, is a PULL towards what you want, how you want to feel and who you want to become, instead of pushing away from what you don't.

If you know you want to feel happy, confident and proud, choose to put your focus and attention on feeling this way and becoming this person. Taking inspired action and making aligned choices will begin to happen easily.

I love lifting weights and have for years and rarely need to feel motivated to get to the gym (except on some really cold, dark winter mornings. I am human, after all, and who doesn't love a warm cozy bed?). I genuinely enjoy my time there and I'm inspired by feeling strong, capable and curious about what I can do. I don't need to motivate myself because I'm not running away from anything, nor is exercise a punishment for the jelly beans I enjoyed last night. I'm not even trying to defy aging! (OK, maybe just a little. . .) I'm simply inspired to feel the way the gym makes me feel.

So often I see women feel like they can't make a positive change in their lives unless they've got something they don't like driving them forward. In between downloading the latest workout craze videos on YouTube to binge on later and bookmarking the hottest new diet tips in their browser, they shame themselves. They constantly beat themselves up for not being good enough.

I want you to flip that around so you understand what it is you really want, unapologetically.

I want you to focus on what you DO want, not on what you don't and what it will take for you to become the person who achieves all of this with ease. Because you can.

When you master this, you'll feel inspired to get up and do the inner and outer work every single day to move forward. No, it's not always easy. It's not always stuff you're going to love. But when you're inspired by what you're going after, you will keep going even through those moments. Let your inner coach keep you going.

Over time, this will result in habit change. Notice I don't say "bad habits" -- it's time to stop the judgment and shame and focus on creating new, healthy ways of thinking and acting.

I want you to figure out what you need to do so that those old habits become less appealing *by default*. How cool does that sound?

When it comes to healthy eating, the E.A.T! Framework will empower you to add nutrients into your daily nutrition plan as opposed to "should-ing" all over yourself and not actually making any changes.

Healthy changes result from healthy choices.

But those healthy choices aren't just about the food you put in your body. It's the thoughts you think and the choices you make to support your transformation from the inside out.

What activities do you love to do that make you feel great about yourself? Choose to include more of them in your life to make your inner coach's job even easier.

If you get into a fight with a friend, your kids are driving you crazy or you just want your husband to move to Timbuktu, what can you do to help yourself feel the way you want to feel? How can you react differently by putting the focus on you?

This is where self-care becomes an absolute foundation of your self-love. It's the willingness on your part to allow your feelings to speak for themselves. Take responsibility for what you actually need in order to feel better as opposed to waiting for other people to help you feel better. It's *your* responsibility.

Here's the thing, self-care is not selfish; it is life-giving, the cornerstone of your self-worth, and your "enoughness."

I don't care if you were told otherwise growing up; this is a fundamental belief you need to lean in to. Your health and happiness (and weight loss) depend on it.

If that means you have to write out all of the things that make you feel good, please do so. And make sure you have some quick wins and big rewards on that list! Then when you find yourself in a sticky situation, silence the critic's voice. Take care of yourself by engaging in an activity that makes you feel awesome. It'll feel like you just flipped a switch!

It's okay to give up things that don't serve you -- like running marathons if they require constant motivation to get your feet pounding the pavement.

Think about it; if you don't love doing something, you won't do it well -- especially if you're hard-pressed to make a connection between it and your Why.

This can move you into a vicious cycle of self-judgement, negativity, resentment and anger.

Do the things you love, and you will receive more self-love in return.

When you say NO to something, you open up space to say YES to something else.

Just as this requires you to take responsibility for yourself and your actions, you also have to release responsibility for other people's actions or reactions.

Don't be afraid to start setting boundaries with people, too. Don't be afraid to start saying no to people.

As you continue your transition towards a relationship with food and your body that you love, you'll start to realize how important to your mental and emotional health boundary setting is.

Are you a caretaker? Are you a people-pleaser? Are you a control freak? What things do you need to start saying no to?

Maybe you can start asking for help. Shocking, I know! But things *can* get done without you doing everything.

In what areas of your life do you need to ask for help?

Instead of driving your kids everywhere, how can you get other people to help? How can you empower them to find their own rides if they're old enough? Where else can your kids and husband help out? Laundry, dishes or dare I say the shopping?

Letting go can feel uncomfortable. Remember, you're working with your resistance, and I promise even if they don't do it as well as you would; done is better than perfect.

If you're a yes-person but you're tired and exhausted and drained, you have permission to be with the uncomfortable emotions that come up when you say, "NO!"

I bet just thinking about saying that 2-letter word makes you squirm. After all, what will *they* think if you say no?

That's what setting boundaries is all about. Boundaries are a self-care tool that aren't about keeping people out, but allowing more of *you* into your own schedule and life. You can't save someone dying of thirst with an empty bucket! And we can't truly be there for the people we love if we're saying yes to everything and everyone except ourselves.

The airplane rule of putting your oxygen mask on yourself first before other people applies to your own thoughts as well. You have to be able to put yourself at the top of your own pile.

This is how you're going to unravel that negative relationship with food. By just being with your emotions and coaching yourself, you will no longer need food to soothe yourself. Healthy boundaries will keep others from infringing on your journey to stay inspired.

So listen to your coach.

Put that oxygen mask on.

And just. . . *Breathe.*

PROGRESS NOT PERFECTION

Our internal dialogue fueled by our beliefs is how we hold ourselves back from achieving lasting weight loss. You can't have a body you love if you're constantly berating it. You'll never let yourself achieve lasting weight loss without permanently silencing your critic and anchoring in new ways of thinking and feeling about your body and food.

Start by listing out all the negative thoughts you have about your body.

Write out 5 things you want to become the new beliefs about your body.

Pick the one belief you want the most and write it in an "I AM" statement on your bathroom mirror.

Write it daily in your journal, repeat it to yourself in the mirror and end your day anchoring in this truth. Feel it in your bones and hammer it home until it becomes the truth.

Fight for who you want to become and you'll disempower your critic.

Chapter 5
The E.A.T! Framework (And the Story Behind It)

Did you know that there is such a thing as "Dieters Anonymous"?

If our exploration of dopamine, serotonin and oxytocin in Chapter 2 didn't do the trick to make the connection between addiction and emotional eating, this fact just about takes the cake!

In the Introduction, you learned why a diet plan without a mindset change is a recipe for struggle and suffering. What works for a celebrity or supermodel may not work for you because you're not them -- and they're not you.

When my husband entered rehab, I had to learn all about addiction and the behaviours that drive it. Through that experience, I realized that food is a tool we often use to numb ourselves -- more specifically, the emotions we'd rather not deal with.

What empowered my hubby to get clean and stay clean was his own customized plan, designed according to his needs.

Again, you may not consider yourself a food addict, but the principle still applies. The E.A.T! Framework puts you in charge of a personalized plan to have a healthy relationship with food for the rest of your life.

Yes, this is worlds apart from the usual dietary advice you've probably been getting for awhile. In my client Paulette's case, we had to release *years* of indoctrination about what was "good" for her.

"You recognize where people are at and try to work with that. This is different than what I have been told for years. I feel great and never deprived."

Remember, this work is not about following trends or one-size-fits-all meal plans. This is all about *you*. *You* decide what you want to eat based on how *you* want to feel. *You* get to check in with *your* body and feel how different foods impact *your* mood.

Not only will the E.A.T! Framework teach you the specifics of protein, carbohydrates and fats, but I also focus heavily on a choice mindset. There is no room for deprivation when you embrace this principle (Chapter 6).

The fact is, writing about how to eat healthy is the easiest part of my job. The true transformation comes when you learn what works for your body ·· and why ·· and how to personalize the Framework.

Want to eat paleo? Go right ahead. All about gluten-free living? Be my guest.

That's the point of a Framework, really. In fact, I used to call it the E.A.T! *System* until a live coaching call last year.

During the group session, an "Aha!" moment followed by an "Oh, shit!" moment came when I realized that no 2 clients had personalized E.A.T! in the same way.

Some women love a good steak while others turn their noses up at any mention of red meat. Some have sensitivities to gluten while others can eat a sandwich and still feel like a million bucks.

The problem with a system is that it's a rigid structure. A set of elements that work together in the same way every time.

If E.A.T! fit *that* definition of a system, it would work for probably fewer than one percent 1% of my clients. But E.A.T! gets results for 9 out of every 10 people because it's flexible and adjustable.

What I teach is just the essentials and how they work to support individual needs -- this is literally the definition of a framework!

The new name stuck.

It totally makes sense as the E.A.T! framework because no single food affects 2 people in the exact same way. Again, my beef with the so-called experts in the diet industry is their objective to push their agenda without helping anyone understand the science behind what they eat.

Tania's words say it best.

"People will tell you, 'It's easy to lose weight, just eat fruits and vegetables', 'Don't eat so much' and 'Count calories'. E.A.T! is more than that. It's the science behind food, it's the science of combining foods. It's also getting to the bottom of what's really stopping you from getting you where you want to be. This has been more than just food, this has been about finding out the reasons behind my poor choices and binging."

If only I could fit all of that on a billboard! I love Tania's attitude because nowhere in her experience was there a hint of deprivation or obsessive self-denial. Eating should be about what you CAN eat, not what you can't!

I want you focused on abundance and all the amazing things that you can eat while still making amazing changes to your body and creating a better lifestyle for you and your family.

Imagine that, focusing on abundance while losing weight. This is how you ditch dieting for good. Even when you make mistakes, it's not the end of the world.

I'll prove it to you.

A couple of years ago, I attended a real estate agent awards dinner with my husband. At the upscale hotel, a gorgeous buffet of food sat spread out, welcoming guests with tantalizing treats both salty and sweet.

The chocolate ganache cake was THE. BEST. that evening. Absolutely divine -- so light it almost floated into my mouth.

Of course, I don't eat desserts like that on a day-to-day basis. I don't have chocolate cake lying around my house!

After enjoying every last bite -- including the crumbs -- of my slice, I noticed the waiter moving table to table.

Plate after plate of chocolate cake, he picked up. The other guests were "finished." Two nibbles of frosting and you're done? Really?

Most of the other women at my table knew that I was a fitness coach (and previously a fitness competitor) and that I knew more about nutrition than most physicians.

Yet none of them followed my lead by partaking in the chocolate decadence set in front of us. They suffered through one tiny mouthful before pushing it around their plates with a fork like toddlers.

If you're going to eat something, *eat it.*

I could almost hear these women's inner dialogue.

"Oh, I shouldn't be eating this. This isn't good for me. This isn't part of my diet. Lucky her that she can eat whatever. I'm gaining weight just looking at this."

The truth I recognized that night -- the one those self-shaming and self-guilting women didn't -- was too simple.

That single piece of chocolate cake was not going to make a difference in my life 5 years later, much less 2 hours after I ate it.

The cake wouldn't have an impact on my body because of how I eat and the choices I make day to day.

Bottom line? I was able to eat it and move on. No guilt, no shame and NO regret. Decisions about what I want to eat are never, "Should I?" or "Shouldn't I?" but simply, "Do I want to eat this? Yes or no?"

I make my choice, own my decision and *move the hell on.* And to be clear, I wasn't in the gym the next day doing extra cardio to compensate.

I'm sharing this with you because this mindset and lifestyle is available to you. I'm not some special snow-flake with a unique metabolism. When you change how you think and feel about food and your body and instead make choices from a place of empowerment, the freedom you're seeking will be yours.

That's the beauty of the E.A.T! framework. You don't have to be riddled with judgment or shame or guilt! You can simply eat what you want to eat and then move on with your life. When you understand how to eat better most of the time -- and I will show you exactly how -- you can have the chocolate cake without a single second guess.

My client Jessie had a very similar experience after enjoying more comfort foods than she typically chooses to allow herself.

But instead of staring in the mirror after coming home and cursing herself, she saw the same truth I did.

"I returned home from a trip with a few extra pounds but am not worried because the E.A.T! course has taught me a better way to eat."

Thanks to the E.A.T! framework, Jessie has educated herself about what healthy choices look like for *her.* She's taken action, and she's seen the results.

That's partially what the E.A.T! acronym stands for, by the way -- Education, Action, Transformation.

When it comes to the Education piece, you deserve to know that although all calories count, not all calories are created equal. There's a very big difference between eating healthy, and eating to change your body composition or lose weight.

My client Lindsay knew all about the eating healthy part, which is why she was skeptical at first about E.A.T! but after learning about eating for *her* body -- not anyone else's -- she very much changed her tune.

"Sometimes the foods you think are healthy might actually be what are holding your body back from making significant changes. Within a week, I saw changes in my body, and I loved that I had energy all day. I was NEVER hungry!"

Those women at the real estate dinner probably thought they were eating healthy by limiting themselves to a few licks of icing. But the fact is, you're not going to feel better, look better or have a better understanding of how to feed your family if you see food as "good" or "bad."

Own your choices without judgment, shame or guilt.

Own your cake.

PROGRESS NOT PERFECTION

With the E.A.T! framework, you will say goodbye to deprivation and the feelings of self-loathing that usually come with it.

To prepare for abundant living and eating, "clean your plate" of previous diets or nutrition plans that didn't work out. When did you feel deprived, and what did you feel coerced into giving up?

Reflecting on the past allows you to experience freedom in the present -- and enjoy a satisfying, fulfilling, deprivation-free future.

ON PREVIOUS DIETS, I FELT DEPRIVED WHEN. . .

Chapter 6
Fit Mind, Fit Body

The year was 2007.

I'd broken the top 10 at the Fitness Universe Pageant in Miami with the best of the best in fitness. After 7 years and numerous top ranking finishes, this was by far the most thrilling moment of my competitive journey.

At any rate, I was fit. Really, *really* fit.

As you can imagine, women all over my city ·· and all over the internet ·· came to me asking for advice.

After saying, "Wow, I could NEVER look like that!" they'd ask me with a straight face, "Can you help me look like that?"

Our words always give away our beliefs.

Before I found my passion in the world of fitness and nutrition, I didn't think of myself as a "healthy" person. I'd certainly never been overweight and had grown up dancing, but the truth is, I never really loved my body. What can I say; I was a junk food junkie! I loved microwave popcorn and sugary Slurpees. I even *smoked*.

My parents took very good care of us and provided us with solid nutrition, but I somehow found myself captive to cravings at a young age. I can still remember eating Rice Krispies with a layer of sugar sprinkled on top. I always found euphoria at the bottom of the bowl when all that was left was milk and sugar!

I also used to sneak sugar cubes from my dad's office and eat the iced tea mix right out of the container.

Hell yes, it's gross to even think about now! But back then, it was absolute *bliss*.

After my second pregnancy, I decided I wanted to make a change -- a BIG change. I successfully grew my fitness coaching business, but I knew that if I wanted to get amazing results for my clients, it had to start with me.

If *my* mindset around eating didn't change, I knew theirs wouldn't either.

A few weeks into our work together, I saw my clients make greater strides in terms of getting stronger and feeling better, but many weren't seeing the body composition changes they expected.

I'd ask a few casual questions about their average protein intake or their ratio of simple to complex carbs per meal.

Their answers confirmed my suspicion.

Clients who understood the role nutrition played in weight loss got the results they wanted.

But clients who didn't understand the role nutrition played -- or worse, *misunderstood* it -- just got frustrated.

All of these women wanted to lose weight, but I soon realized the key was their mindset around what they put into their bodies. Many didn't realize that their breakfast had a bigger impact on how they looked and how they felt than how many reps they did!

I decided it was time for me to see what I could do to change my own body composition. I'm very much a hands-on learner, so I bounced back and forth between some very good fitness and nutrition coaches (and some very bad ones) 'til I found what worked for me.

One of my first coaches had me eating nothing but white fish, yams and spinach for 6 weeks. Coupled with diuretics, this is an example of what NOT to do. I did get lean, but I felt like shit! Not a lifestyle I could or would sustain.

However, that deprivation-driven diet did spark my fascination with how much my body composition could change, and I decided I needed to learn more. It made sense to enter fitness competitions and seek out more qualified coaches. Soon, my love of junk food had been replaced by a love for how my body started to look and feel. I found the knowledge I needed to better support my own clients.

Interestingly enough, deprivation diets like fish and yam were all too common backstage, I later found out. Women who looked like they walked off the cover of fitness magazines were not at all happy with their bodies.

Here they were, looking flawless, and their secret to so-called "success" was constant deprivation and misery around food. Their complaints were the same as the normal women who came to me as clients.

The beta version of the E.A.T! Framework actually came out of my desire to marry the two worlds -- no-deprivation nutrition and body composition change.

Yes, drastically changing your body composition is possible without depriving yourself. Of course, I learned this only *after* firing the yam coach and working with a different mentor who "got" it. She taught me that I didn't need to starve myself along the way. Discipline was required to create an elite physique, but never deprivation.

And I've been teaching other women to "get it" ever since.

Even after having a third son, I've not gone back to the days of living in a place of lack. I love candy, I love ice cream and I especially love my double bubble bubble-gum, but I've learned how to work with my cravings and my choices.

See? It's completely FINE to be open about the foods you love. There's no shame for you to feel that way about the foods you love either.

I don't want to be that person who publicly judges and shames others while I have this deep, dark secret struggle I'm ashamed of.

Living with integrity means being honest with your-self first.

My friend Nari, a Doctor of Naturopath, pointed that out when I asked her about her experience with the E.A.T! Framework.

"Lisa lives honestly and with integrity. You don't see her preaching one thing then doing the other. She has high standards but teaches us how to do that because she does it herself."

But at the end of the day -- and the end of this book, for that matter -- the E.A.T! Framework is not about my mindset, it's all about YOUR mindset.

Are you ready to take responsibility for how you want to feel? Are you ready to be *selfish* about how you want to feel?

I know it sounds strange, but if we can't be selfish about how we want to feel about ourselves and in our lives, nobody else is going to come down with a magic wand and hand that to us. Taking responsibility for how you want to feel (and being selfish about how you want to feel) is a grand act of self-care and self-love.

The best relationship we need to have in this world is the one we have with ourselves. When we are tending to how we want to feel -- when we are even *selfish* about it -- everybody around us benefits.

We have better relationships with our friends, our chil-dren, our spouses and our colleagues. It all comes back to feeling great about ourselves. We are much more pleasant to be around, and we're able to give more and spread that positive energy around.

Your success at this is 100% percent dependent on you. That's what I learned very quickly in my competition days. No coach could get me from point A to point B if I wasn't willing to show up, do the work and keep showing up. Consistency is one of the many keys of success.

The next few chapters in particular are going to be the most information-dense of the book when it comes to nutrition. You're going to go back to school to learn about food, and we're going to strip down everything you think you know to build from the ground-up again.

I really, really encourage you to take in the information and implement it as we go -- ideally, one week at a time.

As we go through each layer of your Nutritional Blueprint, it's imperative that you do your best to stay in the game and support yourself.

The food choices you do or do not make in the days and weeks ahead, do not impact the size or shape of my body. This is all about YOU. Again, I'm not here to wag my finger at you, try to make you feel ashamed or guilty or treat you like you've done something bad. Food is neutral. It really is.

I want you to learn how to celebrate your own successes, even if it's the smallest thing, from choosing to have a healthy salad at lunch instead of having a side of fries or only eating one cookie instead of the box.

SO many weight loss programs are driven by somebody else giving you positive or negative feedback. But what you're learning in this book and the E.A.T! Framework is that only YOU are responsible for giving yourself daily positive feedback. It's part of your successful weight loss mindset and is non-negotiable if you want to achieve phenomenal results.

The fact is, no amount of clean eating will change your weight or body composition if your mindset doesn't change first. I've seen this over and over again with women who have NO CLUE that when they're criticizing their bodies, they're not in alignment with their intentions.

Their health changed little because their thinking changed little.

The sad part is, these women also believed that if they just got that excess weight off, then they would be happy. Then their lives would be complete. The truth is, it's got to be about more than that. Weight loss is an emotional journey. You have to change what's going on between your ears if you're going to ever have lasting transformation.

If you don't believe you can, if you're not ready to make the changes you need to make, nothing is going to happen. As the saying goes, "If you think you can, you will; and if you think you can't, you won't."

So you can *say* you want weight loss until you're blue in the face, but pay attention to what your stories are about what it takes to lose weight. What are you stories about healthy eating and dieting?

What are you willing to become? *Who* are you willing to become?

What does that fit, healthy person look like? What stereotype have you attached to them? And are you willing to let go of those stereotypes and give yourself permission to step into what you want?

You can't become what you're resentful of.

If you're unwilling to take the emotional journey that's tied to your relationship with food, you will always struggle with keeping weight off.

I know because I've worked with women who've lost weight a gazillion times, then put it right back on a gazillion times. This is their missing piece. They haven't done the powerful mindset work that is going to create lasting results.

For example, maybe you believe that you're really lazy when it comes to food. What if you're not lazy, but use that as an excuse because you're not comfortable with cooking? It's normal for us to create stories to hide what we're not as willing to look at.

Are you willing to reframe the type of person that you want to be to achieve the outcome you desire?

Think about what you need to do to change that persona; a lazy person isn't going to get where they want to in life. As long as you continue to believe that about yourself, you're perpetuating the story and you won't take the action that you need to take.

Personally, I've had to change the way I think about money. My relationship with it made it very, very hard to grow my business. Think about it. I thought that having money meant you were a greedy person who wasn't nice to others!

How could I possibly allow abundance to come into my business if I believed that having money was horrible and would make me a horrible person?

I wanted more of it but -- in the same breath -- would curse it. I resented it, hated it. I believed that if I didn't have to deal with it and I didn't have my debt, life would be coming up roses. Nothing could have been further from the truth.

We block the things we want from ever reaching us because of the beliefs we have about them.

So look at what you believe you have to do in order to create what you want for yourself. And then ask if it's true. Chances are, it's not. You can become anything you want to be.

When you become conscious of the beliefs you have and the thoughts you think, you can change how you feel. And when you think and feel differently, you make different choices. Voilà, you've just created an entirely new (and outrageously awesome) outcome.

This is YOUR journey. Make choices that support how you want to feel. They *will* move you forward in the direction of your dreams. Again, caring for yourself is not self indulgent, it is the cornerstone of survival and the foundation of your self worth.

My client Stacey lost 16 pounds and 16 inches in just 12 weeks in part because of the role that self care played in her life.

"Taking time for myself to be happy and health is okay," she shared with me.

Stacey changed her story, which changed her mindset, which changed her weight.

That's exactly what I want for you, too.

PROGRESS NOT PERFECTION

Shame has no place in self care, just as deprivation has no place in creating a healthy relationship with food.

We can release our shame when we name it, claim it and make the choice to no longer allow ourselves to believe the story that fuels it.

Shame is the belief that we are defective. It's a focus on self. Its effects are self loathing, feelings of inferiority and persistent thoughts that you don't measure up. Shame is behind behaviours such as isolation and anything that hides our insecurities, embarrassment or humiliations.

Guilt, on the other hand, is a focus on behaviour and helps us to course correct. Guilt allows us to make amends, admit our mistakes and look to improve. In dieting, people often confuse feelings of shame, believing it's just guilt they're experiencing. It's important that you recognize the difference, or shame will continue to hold you hostage.

To change your mindset, you must change how you think and feel about yourself by becoming the person who feels good in her body, has gratitude for its gifts, has a healthy relationship with food and no longer allows shame to play a role in her life.

In the space provided below, I want you to create the woman you want to become.

We can't create in our minds what's not possible in real life. Where do you think the first idea for flight, space travel and the iPhone came from?

Each of these started with the courage to imagine and believe in what was possible BEFORE it became a reality.

This is the visioning process for lasting weight loss and permanent mindset shifts that create a peaceful and fulfilling relationship with both food and your body.

How does she feel about her body?

What kind of clothes does she wear?

What does she say to herself when she looks in the mirror?

What kind of activities does she love?

How does she feel about herself in her life?

What does she love to do?

What things does she do to take care of herself?

How does she feel about food?

How does she make choices?

What things would she say to herself if she ate cookies?

What would be important to her?

What things would she say yes to?

What would she say no to?

What would a normal day look like in her world?

What thoughts would she think?

What mantras would she have?

What would she believe to be possible?

What would get her excited?

How would her life be different from how you're living now?

How would she celebrate herself?

What kind of people is she surrounded by?

What are her relationships with others like?

How does she define success?

Chapter 7
The Nutrition Your Body Is Asking For

"Change."

Ask a thousand people what metabolism is, and nobody will probably answer with that word. But that's exactly what the word originally meant!

Really, metabolism is just a fancy way of describing how foods change when they enter your body. Your metabolism is measured by the rate at which your body burns through the food you put into it.

We've all heard the phrase "fat burning"; THAT is what your metabolism is responsible for.

When you're feeding your body at regular intervals throughout the day, your body is going to be forced to break down those foods faster and burn through them.

Starving yourself is the most effective way to NOT lose weight! If you're having significant periods of time where you go without eating, your body slows down your metabolism.

Your body is designed to survive and will do everything it needs to maintain life. If your body thinks you're trying to starve it to death, it goes into protection mode.

It's a similar response to what would happen if you jumped into a frozen lake; in order to preserve life, your body would automatically slow your heart rate and respiration.

The science of evolutionary biology shows us that in the deep human past, there were regular famines. Before agriculture, the only plants in your diet were those you found growing in the wild, and the only meat you could sink your teeth into belonged to animals your tribe could kill.

Life was rough, to say the very least. Over eons, our bodies evolved to conserve energy. You could even say our bodies are designed by nature to store fat!

So if you want to speed up your metabolism, don't communicate to your body that there's a famine when there is not. Eat at regular intervals throughout the day. This is the key to long-term body composition change.

I like to talk to my clients about these regular intervals using medieval terms.

"Breakfast like a *king*, lunch like a *prince* and dinner like a *pauper*."

Eat the bulk of your calories earlier in the day, taper off around mid-day and ease off into the evening.

This approach flies in the face of the popular "skip breakfast" and "fast all the time" diet advice you may have heard.

So think about WHY you would do it differently. Shouldn't you match how much you eat with how active you are during the day?

Most people are super busy in the morning. By bed time, they've put their feet up after the kids have fallen asleep.

Time your caloric intake around your energy output.

It's a simple rule, but it works. Make nature your ally, not your enemy.

But how easy is it to flip this picture? In our Netflix and Hulu culture, we flip on the television and binge on junk shows and junk food. If you skipped the meals your body needed, you'll find your hand in a bag of Cheetos while watching the *Gilmore Girls* reboot.

If only we listened to what our bodies are trying to tell us! Hunger cues throughout the day are teachable moments from Mother Nature that most of us ignore.

First thing in the morning, it's easier to throw back a cup of your favorite java than have a proper breakfast. *Caffeine in hand, and off you go!*

Then when you start to feel the rumbling, you down another cup at work without paying attention to the message behind your mood.

Over time, we desensitize ourselves to our bodies' requests. We seem to be the only animal on the planet that's forgotten how to eat! We've overridden our bodies' wisdom by following someone else's diet plan. We've become more interested in eating what's convenient than in nurturing our bodies.

The message of hunger is a plea for a nutritious meal, but we choose to down a few gulps of appetite-suppressing caffeine instead so we can get on with our day.

Your body KNOWS what it needs to eat because it's trying to support your life! That also means you have to pay attention to how you're feeling and stop making your body's needs anything less than a priority.

We've also run into a problem with portion distortion. Over the years, the size of our plates and serving sizes have grown. When I was a kid, a small fry at McDonald's was actually, you know. . .*small*. Fast forward a few years, and the large fry my parents used to split with us kids is the new small!

We don't need larger portions; we need smaller portions spread throughout the day.

You're either nodding with an internal knowing as you're reading these statements, or your mind is being blown by these truths for the first time.

Somewhere along our food journey, we've learned behaviours that aren't good for our bodies. They keep us stuck in the status quo. Most of us know what we should be doing. . .but just don't.

Before you breeze from this sentence to the next, ask yourself this question, then pause 'til your body gives you the honest answer.

Do I actually eat when I'm hungry? Or do I eat when I feel like it?

The two are very different. Maybe that emotional eating pattern appears spontaneously when you're feeling sad. Maybe you had a fight with your husband or your kids.

Past stories drive how you relate to food now, too.

Did you grow up in a family where you were made to stay at the table until you finished everything on your plate?

Was your mom constantly harping on you to not waste food?

As you recognize those stories and beliefs, ask yourself if the behaviour patterns they created are serving you. Are you really hungry, or did you just get triggered because your kids are wasting food?

Here in North America, we have an incredible amount of abundance that other parts of the world simply do not. In spite of that abundance, we're eating like we're in lack!

If you feel guilty about throwing out food because your body tells you it's satisfied, get curious about where that belief originated from and decide if it's still serving you.

If you're really concerned and want to make a difference to those who aren't as fortunate, please donate to UNICEF or another organization that feeds children around the world.

I guarantee that you cleaning your plate does not save someone who is starving elsewhere in the world. All you end up doing is perpetuating your own sense of lack, which leads to overeating and puts you in the state of not being loving or caring for your body.

Speaking of first world abundance, we have clean water within arm's reach for the majority of our day. Yet somehow, we're constantly dehydrated! According to a survey by the Nutrition Information Center, 75% of Americans are *chronically* dehydrated. Clearly, this isn't good! No wonder we feel lethargic all the time.

The fact is, because our bodies are made mostly of water molecules, we operate better when we're properly hydrated. We sleep better, too. In fact, fatigue is an indicator of dehydration in many cases.

Just as your smartphone is within a few meters of you at all times, keep a water bottle nearby as well. It's easy to build new habits when you just add another task to one that already comes second-nature to you.

So to get the 2 to 3 liters of water your body needs everyday, make sure that a water bottle is as close to you as your cell phone is.

And instead of chowing down on a few huge meals in the afternoon, pace yourself and graze throughout the day, enjoying 4 or 5 smaller meals. Drink at least 2 glasses of water during each meal, and your body will get the hydration it needs.

Whether it's drinking more water or dining on frequent portions throughout the day, the more you pay attention to what your body needs, the more clearly it will communicate its needs to you.

When we tune out that communication, the consequences are way worse than just bad cravings.

One client of mine, Lorelei, found herself diagnosed with Colitis before she was 40. A combination of stress and unhealthy diet made her body give off warning signs, but like so many of us, she didn't know how to listen to her own body.

Attacks of pain lasted anywhere from 6 to 8 weeks. Colon polyps appeared. Her body lost the ability to absorb nutrients from her GI tract for good.

Her risk of cancer more than doubled every single year she suffered symptoms. This was really scary stuff!

But when she adopted the E.A.T! Framework you're learning, everything turned around. Lorelei chose to listen to her body's needs, and she's been attack-free for over 24 months and counting.

The weird thing is, Lorelei *thought* she was okay. . .before everything went sour, that is.

Another client, Jane, called out this irony, "What we are told by mainstream media is really not accurate – so many of us 'think' we eat healthy based on the information we are fed through these mediums."

To put it another way, we think we're eating healthy until our bodies show us otherwise. I'm just glad that Lorelei got ahold of E.A.T! before it was too late.

I held nothing back in the introduction when I targeted the diet fads and nutrition trends. Food manufacturers absolutely do NOT have our best interest in mind!

Let's back away from the hype, put down the lifestyle magazines, unsubscribe from the hot new fitness blog, and keep it simple.

If it walks on the earth, flies in the sky, swims in the ocean, grows in the ground or comes off a tree or bush, you can eat it.

There. That's all the nutrition you need to know. For now, at least.

Creating a better relationship with food always brings you back to the basics.

That's why I love a short list of ingredients, which I'll give you at the end of this chapter. If you have to twist your tongue into a knot to pronounce the ingredients on a label, put that shit back on the shelf!

The healthiest foods for us are NOT those with the bright labels with symbols everywhere screaming how healthy they are. A potato is just a potato. No fanfare needed. Healthy doesn't get any simpler than this.

Yet we question, we fear, we look for better manmade solutions because of what some diet touted back in the 80's. Most women I talk to STILL think eating potatoes will make them fat.

If you take one look at many of these healthier options with their health check symbols and low-fat and sugar-free labels, you'll realize that the marketing minds behind them are just trying to manipulate you into believing their foods are super-healthy for you.

They even manipulate serving sizes. At first glance, a food may look low-calorie, low-carb or low-fat, but in truth, they're just hooking you to buy. I mean seriously, who only eats 5 crackers?

So don't buy the hype. One look at the ingredient list and serving size breakdown will tell you everything that the flashy product packaging does not.

It's your job to decide whether or not you want to put

something in your body. You're the one in control, not some food CEO who's only objective is to increase his bottom line -- not shrink yours.

Only YOU can determine what foods will help you look, feel and perform your best.

And I'm here to help you make those informed decisions.

You cannot unknow what you now know.

PROGRESS NOT PERFECTION

Is your kitchen ready to E.A.T.?

Choosing nutritious foods without having to think twice about it requires a supportive environment in your home. Don't keep that extra chocolate bar in the back of the freezer and lie to yourself, "Well, I just won't eat it."

We both know you will.

Don't play the willpower game. I have many times, and I always lose. If you want something, go and have it, but put your butt in the car and drive yourself to get it. But you do not need to keep it in your house.

Instead, get your kitchen ready for your new lifestyle -- one where you're always empowered to make the right food choices for *your* body, even if you don't wake up with the willpower of a professional fitness pro.

STOCK YOUR KITCHEN WITH THE FOLLOWING FOODS:

- ☐ Extra Lean Beef
- ☐ Wild Caught Fish
- ☐ Chicken
- ☐ Eggs and Egg Whites
- ☐ Balsamic Vinegar
- ☐ Olive Oil
- ☐ Flax Oil
- ☐ Almonds
- ☐ Natural Peanut Butter
- ☐ Wild Rice
- ☐ Quinoa
- ☐ Steel Cut Oatmeal
- ☐ Yams
- ☐ Sweet Potato
- ☐ Wild Rice
- ☐ Raw Nuts
- ☐ Fruit (Variety)
- ☐ Vegetables (5 Kinds, 2 of Which Must Be   Dark Green)
- ☐ Turkey
- ☐ Edamame

Chapter 8
The Past, the Present and the Power of Food Logs

By the time many women start a new diet, they're convinced it will work just as well as the last one did.

And that one didn't.

I recently had a client show resistance to letting go of what she'd done in the past to lose weight.

"But it worked," she claimed.

I gently but firmly showed her it didn't. If it had, she wouldn't STILL be seeking a solution.

Lo and behold, the weight was back, and she was about to repeat the same cycle.

We've all heard the quote, "The definition of insanity is doing the same thing over and over hoping for different results."

Just because you lost weight doesn't mean the diet worked.

It didn't.

I see this attitude over and over in my work, whether it's a 20-something girl training for a marathon or a middle aged mother of 5 who wants to finally say goodbye to the baby weight.

You've come to me for a reason. But if you've got one foot in the past, you'll sabotage yourself.

Quite often as human beings, we look to our past to predict our future. We just can't help it.

Did the last diet work? No. So what's probably going to happen with this new one?

The truth is, we can't predict our future any more than we can go into the past and rewrite what happened.

How many diets have you tried? How many times have you lost the weight, then gained it back a few weeks later? How many face-down moments have you had? How many tears and tantrums have you gone through?

These are painful questions, I know. But the answers are not weapons to beat yourself up. Experience is not a compass for the journey ahead.

Reflecting on the past is not the same thing as looking to the past like it's a crystal ball. Be mindful of what's happened before, but keep your eyes forward.

I've stumbled and fallen a gazillion times, and I always get back up. Before working on my mindset, I'd get back up but be so attached to my past experiences that I felt paralyzed when trying to move forward. I was afraid of making mistakes, falling down yet again and feeling disappointed.

I'm sure you can relate as you reflect on your weight loss journey up to this point. I had to shift my mindset and learn that my face-down moments had absolutely NO impact on what was possible in the future unless I gave them meaning.

Imagine starting every day with a blank slate, full of opportunity and possibility.

This isn't a pipe dream.

It's the truth.

Now, I know where the future is. And it's not behind me. Now, I don't let past failures -- learning experiences or whatever the hell you want to call them -- colour my choices today or tomorrow.

That can be incredibly difficult, especially when you've experience disappointment in yourself before. Nobody wants to feel discouraged, like they've failed and it's all their fault.

That's why we try to use the past as a predictor for the future, to prepare us for yet another let-down. How sick and twisted is that?

So what if your new eating plan doesn't work out!

And what if it does?

"But you don't know my story, Lisa!" I had one elderly woman break down into tears in my studio. "I've been fat since your grandparents were in school."

I wonder how many years she beat herself up with that self-hate.

What if she'd quit using her past as a frame of reference 30 years ago?

What if she'd stopped making her weight mean something about her identity?

Her story would have played out very differently, I'm sure.

You don't have to follow her example though. If you start fresh today without looking at your future through the lens of the past, what would you do differently?

What choices would you make? What programs would you jump into? Who would you decide to work with? Who would you be?

Honestly, I would choose to never go on another diet that makes me feel like I've come down with the flu! Isn't it crazy what passes for "healthy" these days? Opposite-land has never had more citizens, I tell you.

When you see food differently, free from the decisions you've made in the past, you can answer the "What if this works?" question with a healthy sense of optimism.

My client Nancy went through a total physical transformation once she stopped cursing herself for past mistakes -- and the diets she followed that caused her to make them.

She's let go of her own filter, too, which makes me chuckle every time she tells her story.

"Before Lisa, I had never been on a 'diet' that didn't make me feel like shit both physically and psychologically. I am thankful for your balanced approach to eating right and eating healthy. You have helped me see food in a whole new way. Not only do I not feel hungry, I feel energized. Most importantly, I am incredibly appreciative of all your support and encouragement during this journey. Weight and body image issues expose some parts of our psyche that are raw and vulnerable. You have made this journey an easier ride."

The subtext of Nancy's story is my life motto: *Progress, not perfection.*

That woman gets it -- there's no place to get to, there is no "done."

A lifestyle is never "done."

Whether it's a past we feel ashamed of or a future we hope to be completely different, where ever we put our attention and intention expands.

I see too often women stalling their own progress after a few weeks of eating healthy because they almost expect to fail.

Weight Watcher's didn't work. Atkins didn't work. South Beach didn't work. Why would E.A.T!?

They're used to twisting their fork around that last nasty piece of soggy plain spinach. "Eating healthy" is a chore worse than cleaning the bathroom.

In a frat house.

Without gloves.

When treating our bodies with love has become synonymous with feeling disgusted over each meal, there's a problem!

If your attention is on the bad experiences of the past and your intention is to try your hardest until you fail -- again, because that's how it's always been -- the chances of a repeat *skyrocket*.

A few years ago, I made it my intention to travel the world on business. So, I chose to give attention to any opportunities along my path that opened the way for travel.

Just last year, amazing doors opened wide for me -- one to mentor entrepreneurs at a colleague's mastermind retreat in Key West, and St. Pete, Florida, and the other to attend conferences in Laguna Beach and sunny San Diego.

What I focused on, expanded.

As you learn everything you need to know about proteins, carbs and veggies in the coming chapters, remain mindful of where your attention and intention are.

If you've been focused on that number on the scale and all the foods you've had to give up, your attitude will amplify the accompanying emotions. It will feel impossible to lose weight. You'll war with yourself every day over the foods you want to eat. . .but probably shouldn't.

But if you're putting your attention on what you ACTUALLY want for your body -- who you need to become, a new and exciting way to meal plan you can personalize and follow for life -- your relationship with food will change in the *exact* way you want it to.

Every morning when I wake up, I use the acronym "AIR" to get my focus right.

A for attention, I for intention, R for repeat.

Every single day, look at where your attention is.

What are your intentions behind that?

Repeat.

This simple process keeps your focus where it belongs, which is the fastest way to open the door to what you really want for your life, your body and your relationship with food.

When I onboard new students into my 3-day program *No Deprivation Weight Loss*, I start everyone out with a food log. This is the most practical way I know of to change the way you view the past so you can put your attention where it should be going forward.

Instead of beating yourself up because you licked the icing off the cupcake at the party before throwing the rest away, you can remove yourself from the emotional turmoil with a food log.

For that evening, you would write down that you ate a cupcake's worth of chocolate icing -- and that's it! No self-hatred or humiliation.

Like an athlete watching post-game footage of their performance, you can be a witness to exactly what you eat without applying judgment. It's a new kind of consciousness around eating!

A food log is not about "should-ing" all over yourself or restricting your food choices. And it's definitely NOT about judgement, shame or blame. Nor is it about forcing yourself not to eat anything you want to.

Just write down what you eat, and re-read your food log during your Attention, Intention, Repeat practise.

It's a practise to raise your awareness and get conscious about not just your food choices, but the inner dialogue that goes along with them.

If emotion (AKA judgement), swells up for you as you record what you ate and drank today, just be aware of it. Don't run from it or grab a diet root beer on the way to work the next morning to ease away that discomfort.

Food logging is such a powerful exercise because of the clarity it brings to what you're actually eating on a day-to-day basis.

Unconscious eating ends today, and it ends for good.

Once you record your day's food and drink for each meal and the snacks between them (*Progress Not Perfection* section below), you'll become a Nutritional Detective.

Let's get clear on what you're actually putting in your body so it's much, MUCH easier to fill in the gaps.

When I have clients take me through their food logs, I hear feedback like, "Oh, I was surprised how much I was eating," and, "I had no idea how few vegetables I actually ate!"

Being accountable to yourself like this allows you to cultivate trust in your own abilities to make the right choices for you.

When you're eyeing that one thousand calorie sandwich on display at the deli, your immediate thought will be, "Oh, I'm going to have to write that down in my food log. Do I really want to do that?"

Accountability and conscious choice become your sources for empowerment.

As you scan your entries for yesterday, the day before and last week, the key is to not judge or shame yourself for any unhealthy choices. Instead, look at where you're missing the healthy stuff.

A powerful mindset shift occurs when you're able to change your perspective from the negative to look for the wins and the opportunities. Food logs are NOT weapons, but years of dieting have programmed us to loath them instead of embrace the growth they provide.

As you add in the quality nutrients, the cream puffs and sweetened lattes will vanish from your food log over the coming days and weeks.

Another example of growth is to fill in the nutrition gaps you notice in your food logs. *Where are they?*

When reviewing your own food log, start with the protein. Are you including it in every meal? And what does the protein look like?

Then, take those detective skills and look at the timing and number of your meals. Are you eating anywhere from 3 to 5 times a day? How long do you go between eating? Can you shorten those gaps and become a "grazer" to boost your metabolism?

What about the veggies? Are there any vegetables on your food log? I get it, they don't light up your brain chemistry the same way sugar does. But take if from someone with 6-pack abs after 3 pregnancies; nothing makes your body look or feel better than vegetables.

I had to move beyond carrots and broccoli to finally find the veggies that work for me (and that I like). That category definitely doesn't include broccoli -- the stuff tastes like dirt. I don't care how much of a superfood it is, broccoli makes very rare appearances in my food logs because I just don't like it. THIS is the power of choice.

I do eat tons of dark leafy green vegetables -- the power veggies -- like spinach, kale, chard and brussel sprouts.

Those, I like. *The more, the merrier!*

What other colours can you add to your portions of veggies? Yellow peppers and white cauliflower, perhaps?

Just make sure you're getting in your servings every single day (see Chapter 12 for specific recommendations). I see so many people taking green supplements, which are not actual food. They're supplements!

Nothing makes your body look or feel as good as real food does.

Consider your Omega-3 oils as well. For women, managing both carbohydrate cravings and normal hormonal shifts make Omega-3's a necessity. Whether fish or flaxseed oil, Omega-3 oils assimilate so much easier into your body than any other foods do (see Chapter 10 for more about nutritious fats).

Next, look at the setting. No, I don't mean the table setting -- I mean, where the table is set! Have you been eating out? Do you live at restaurants several nights a week?

There is absolutely nothing wrong with eating out. I eat out all the time; I really do enjoy someone bringing me food and cleaning away the dirty dishes afterwards. I have 3 kids after all, so eating out means I can relax and let someone else take care of me, and I'm not having to take care of anybody else.

On menus, learn to look past the chicken strips and french fries. I promise, there's always healthy options if you're willing to look for them. Don't be fooled into thinking salads are the healthy option though. A grilled steak and baked potato can have fewer calories thanks to the cheese, nuts and dressing that get loaded on top of many bowls of iceberg lettuce. Ask questions instead of making assumptions and don't be afraid to make substitutions or special requests.

And how many "fake" foods show up on your logs because you need the convenience? I'm talking bars, shakes, pills, powders or packaged foods. Remember, supplements are just *supplemental* to the real food your body needs.

I get the struggle, of course. We can't always sit down and eat a proper meal. But to feel good in your skin, you have to step back and ask, "Am I important enough to pause for 10 minutes and eat some real food?"

Make yourself a priority. Make sitting down and eating real food your ultimate act of self care. Then, hold yourself accountable to recording everything that makes its way into your mouth.

Like my friend Linda, you'll probably realize after your first few days of food logging, "I thought I ate healthy before."

Because Linda started giving her body the right combination of protein, complex carbs and healthy fats, she's dropped inches and weight and ditched her allergies, insomnia and asthma inhaler.

The fuel we give our body becomes how we feel.

Over the next few chapters, you'll find yourself filling in the nutrition gaps. From proteins and fats to fruit and legumes, your meals will slowly transform from what they have been, to the goal-supporting self-care experiences they should be.

Let's E.A.T!

PROGRESS NOT PERFECTION

For the next 5 days, keep a food log. Track every meal and every snack.

By keeping your focus on how you want to feel, you'll remain accountable to making choices in alignment with that. You'll feel a self-congratulatory rush of joy when you realize that the foods you're logging, will actually help you get where you want to be -- and become the person you want to be.

FOOD LOG: Day #1

FOOD LOG: Day #2

FOOD LOG: Day #3

FOOD LOG: Day #3

FOOD LOG: Day #5

Chapter 9
Your Nutritional Blueprint: Proteins

Anything worth doing well, is worth doing poorly to start.

Remember the time versus intensity chart in Chapter 1?

Most dieters fall flat on their crumb-covered faces into a pile of empty snack wrappers because they try to do everything perfectly from the get-go.

But you're on the path to progress, not perfection. That means I'm not interested in having you live out the remaining days of your life tied to a food scale, nor do I want you counting calories or becoming obsessed with measuring every serving of protein by the gram.

Here's the one caveat:

In order to have this freedom, there IS a learning curve. You can't change what you aren't conscious of, so as you start navigating through E.A.T!, you will need to initially measure and in some cases weigh your food. This is the only way for you to truly know and understand exactly what a serving size looks like for you personally.

The good news is, once you know what your serving sizes look and feel like, you'll be able to go by sight more often than not. If your pants start to feel snug, it's never a bad thing to get yourself in check by measuring and weighing again.

It's easy for my eyes to over-estimate my servings, especially if it's a food I really love. So I make it a practise to weigh and measure my food at least 1 day a month just to stay conscious about my portions. You will soon know the serving sizes of the foods you eat on the regular by heart. And once you know, you cannot unknow.

I have titled this and the following sections of the E.A.T! Framework, "Your Nutritional Blueprint" because of the close relationship between eating well for your body and building a home.

With both, you start out by following blueprints. For your body, consider the E.A.T! Framework your set of plans.

When a new home is constructed, does the builder dismiss the contractors? "Okay, that's a wrap! The house is done. Bring in the demolition crew now to tear this place down!"

Abso-freakin'-lutely not! Yet this is *exactly* what most diets have you do. You follow the plan 'til you're "done," then you stop everything and go back to the way things were before.

Homes are meant to be lived in for decades to come.

The same goes for your own body. Just as breaking a door knob in your home isn't the end of the world, giving into a craving for cheap tacos is nothing to feel ashamed of.

Learning what your body needs in order to THRIVE is like learning anything else, from dancing salsa style to speaking Spanish fluently while doing it.

You're getting the nutritious scoop on proteins FIRST because they're the foundation of your diet, just as concrete is the foundation of a home.

The word protein actually means, "of first importance,"

oddly enough. Yet in our culture of greasy fast food, this macronutrient has vanished from many women's diets.

Protein deficiency, therefore, has become a serious problem. Without enough of it, your body won't be able to form new red blood cells at the rate it needs to, much less create the lean body you'd like to see in the mirror.

Here's the deal; most vegetarian and vegan sources of protein are not true proteins. If it doesn't have a face, more often than not, it's not a true protein.

When making statements like this, I usually get the "stink eye" from all the plant-based eaters in the room.

I get it. There are MANY ways to get from point A to point B, but the E.A.T! Framework supports eating animal-based proteins. If that's not for you, I totally understand. But give yourself permission to be curious as you dive into the next few chapters. You don't know what you might find when you stay open, and I promise, I'm not trying to sell anyone on my way of doing things. I am here to empower you to make the best choices for you!

So let me first clarify what a "true protein" is. It's a protein source that provides a complete amino acid profile. Most are animal-based, but there are two exceptions: edamame (AKA soybeans) and quinoa.

However, due to the breakdown of their protein, carbohydrate and fat ratios, quinoa needs to be treated as a carbohydrate.

Edamame is unique. Technically speaking, edamame is in a category of its own. Its protein and carbohydrate ratio is almost equal, so I have my clients treat it as both. It's the full meal deal and can make a perfect on-the-go snack.

Can you get all the amino acids you need eating plant based proteins? The answer is yes, but it takes education and diligence to understand how to combine different plant-based foods to give your body the complete amino acid profile it requires. These days you can also find many amazing plant based protein supplements on the market to fill the gaps.

If you want to lose weight, animal-based true protein sources are your best friend and greatest ally.

There's a big difference between eating healthy and eating to lose weight. The type of food you put in your body will have a direct impact on how your body looks, feels AND changes shape.

I've often seen women jump into the plant-based food movement because they believe it will be the quickest road to weight loss. But nothing could be further from the truth. Often, they're left wondering how they managed to pack on so many pounds when they were eating "healthy." I promise, we'll dive into this more in the chapters to come.

Here's why understanding the importance of true source proteins in weight loss is so powerful. They are the powerhouse macronutrient that puts your body to work because they require more energy for your body to break down. This process is called *thermogenesis*, and it means your body heats up while you're digesting true protein. Your body is literally burning fat! We're so focused on burning calories in the gym, we've overlooked the calorie-burning process our bodies go through in the process of breaking down and digesting our food!

Think of eating a chicken breast as like slamming your foot on the accelerator of your pickup truck. You're going to zoom past fellow drivers and burn way more fuel than you would driving the speed limit.

But there in the righthand lane is a two-door compact car, slowly putzing along slower than the speed of traffic.

That's like eating legumes. You're still in a vehicle, but you won't get very far very fast.

The difference between animal and plant-based proteins is far from all you need to know to alter your body composition, drop pounds and lose inches.

I classify true proteins into three easy-to-remember groups: lights, mediums and darks. Going by colour and not calorie count makes life SO much easier for all of us!

Light proteins are the leanest. Most have no fat or are very low fat. Think egg whites, chicken breast and turkey breast, raw white fish sushi like tuna, dry cottage cheese curds, white fish and non-fat natural Greek yogurt.

Medium coloured proteins include our friends from the sea, like salmon (cooked or sushi grade), prawns, scallops, crab, sardines and canned tuna. Protein powders that contain a full amino acid profile in their ingredients (both plant based or whey based), as well as a combination whole egg plus egg whites, pork tenderloin, edamame and tofu fit into the medium protein category.

Medium proteins have more fat than light proteins and sometimes arrive on our plates after being processed. Protein powders and canned tuna get marks against them for that reason. Shellfish like shrimp are the dumpsters of the ocean floor, so they're not the highest quality protein out there.

Then we have the dark meats. Most diets will tell you to wrap caution tape around these foods. I'm going to tell you this right now -- dark protein is NOT a crime against nutrition!

The E.A.T! Framework is all about what you *can* eat and how much you *should* eat. The protein layer of the blueprint allows you to choose foods that you love to eat in the right amount.

So if you love beef, bison, chicken and turkey thigh, lamb or servings of two or more whole eggs, that is totally okay. As with carbohydrates (Chapter 11), just stay mindful of how many dark proteins you consume each day.

Speaking of consumption, to implement the E.A.T! Framework for proteins, consume them at EVERY meal.

This means 5 times a day, not 3.

This is the biggest shift for many of my clients. Even if they eat 3 square meals a day and graze in between, they're still not getting enough protein.

Five servings of protein. Grab a pen and scribble that on your wrist if you have to.

Now, take a deep breath.

Progress, not perfection.

If you're only eating 3 meals a day right now, and eating protein 5 times a day seems like too much of a crazy stretch, start where you're at.

Add a protein during those three meals. There's no time limit on getting it right for your body.

To make the next step of progress even easier for you, let me give you a few rules of thumb for white, medium and dark proteins for those 5 servings per day.

The maximum number of light proteins you can have per day is 5. The maximum for medium proteins is 2, and for darks, never more than 1 per day.

The 2-serving maximum for medium proteins comes with one caveat, however. If you eat a whole egg with egg whites for breakfast and shrimp fajitas for lunch, you forfeit the beef ravioli for supper.

To keep this simple, if you have 2 medium proteins in a day, you can kiss your dark serving goodbye until tomorrow.

So if you like to sit down at the dinner table to chow down on chicken thigh or grass-fed steak, manage your lights and mediums throughout the day to make room for that.

This simple protein blueprint really puts the power in your hands.

Notice how little you have to remember: 5, 2, 1. The maximum for lights, mediums and darks.

When it comes to serving size, we don't go back on everything you've learned so far and start you on a formula where you've got to multiply and divide all sorts of numbers.

Start with 2 to 3 ounces of protein per serving, which will give you roughly 15 to 20 grams of protein inside the portion at each meal. There are many factors that determine specific protein requirements, but this is the range that works for the majority of my female clients.

For example, 3 ounces of protein is roughly half of a single chicken breast and contains about 20 grams of protein for that portion.

There's lunch!

See how easy this is?

Stick to that magic number of protein servings per meal, and you're set.

The first layer of your Nutritional Blueprint is now laid.

But proteins aren't the only thing that come from animal products.

Despite the claims of Weight Watchers, you'll learn in Chapter 10 why the next layer of your blueprint is just as important as protein to change your body composition.

Here's a hint -- if you *don't* eat enough of it, your body fat percentage goes up.

The ultimate weight loss paradox awaits you.

PROGRESS NOT PERFECTION

Getting the protein your body needs to kick thermogenesis into high gear as surprisingly easy.

To give yourself 5 different options for eating protein every day, stay mindful of the 5-serving plan below.

For example, you might have egg whites (light) for breakfast, a shrimp salad as a mid-morning snack (medium), chicken breast for lunch (light), Greek yogurt in the afternoon (light) and baked tofu strips (medium) for dinner.

List out your favourite and familiar protein choices below and see how they fit into the E.A.T! Framework as you begin to build out your meals.

YOUR FIVE PROTEIN SERVINGS

- *5 x light*
- *4 x light and 1 x medium*
- *4 x light and 1 x dark*
- *3 x light and 2 x medium*
- *3 x light and 1 x medium and 1 x dark*

Chapter 10
Your Nutritional Blueprint: Fats

"Fat does not make you fat."

Yes, this is the ultimate weight loss paradox.

When I share this strange fact with new clients, many of them give me the look I would expect if I'd just said they don't need oxygen to breathe.

But the skepticism drops like the weight after they've followed their personalized version of the E.A.T! Framework for a few weeks. When those stubborn 5 inches vanish from the tummy, clients cannot help but become true believers!

Some fats actually help your body get leaner quicker and lose weight faster. Surprising, eh?

The best part is, fat is what makes our food taste good -- plain and simple!

As women, when we go on those low-fat diets and remove healthy fats, we put our hormonal health at risk because we leave ourselves in a place of feeling deprived and hungry all the time.

But food manufacturers would rather we *believe* that fat on an ingredient list is the nutritional equivalent of a stop sign.

Truth be told, it's fat in a meal that makes you feel full and satisfied! And if you're full and satisfied, you won't reach for something salty and sweet that's either processed starch or made with high fructose corn syrup.

Like the living legend of entrepreneurship Seth Godin says, "Marketers are liars."

The fact is, fat is ESSENTIAL for a balanced diet.

Now that we've sunk those BS objections to eating it in the first place, let's get specific on which *types* of fat your body needs.

This second layer of your Nutritional Blueprint has a close relationship with the first.

The reason I categorized your protein as light, medium and dark is that there are also residual fats in protein. This allows us to construct healthy boundaries and manage those residual fats. That way, you can add in more healthy fats to promote weight loss. You'll find these residual fats almost everywhere, and I want you to pay attention to them outside of your proteins.

When you're reading labels for condiments, dressing or even in your cooking, make sure you're keeping them under 5 grams of fat per serving. I'm not concerned with trace amounts of fat in food, but if you're choosing a salad dressing with 15 grams of fat in 1 tablespoon, then you're going to have a problem.

This is probably counter-intuitive if you've been hopping on and off the low-fat diets for the past couple of decades. Even just 10 years ago, the belief was that if we stripped fats from our food, everybody would lose weight and get healthier overnight.

But with millions of people now feeling hungry after a low-fat meal, simple sugars and artificial sweeteners appeared on our plates.

And we all know how that ended. The obesity problem became an epidemic because the so-called "experts" stole the second most vital macronutrient from our diets.

Whether you can relate to the low-fat diet struggle or not, I'm here to equip you with the knowledge about fats that leads to greater fat-burning, tissue and nerve healing, more energy, mood improvement, better skin, hair and nail appearance and hormone regulation.

If you suffer from PMS or mood swings, especially in the winter months when most of us don't get enough sunlight, make sure you have your Omega-3's handy.

I've actually had clients come back after taking that advice to tell me, "My PMS symptoms have subsided!"

And let's not forget the power they have to diminish carbohydrate cravings, too.

Before I get into the difference between Omega-3, Omega-6 and Omega-9 fats, be cautious of using them to cook. They're sensitive to heat -- all except coconut oil. Every fat has a different burn point, but your Omega-3's like fish and flax oil absolutely CANNOT be heated, so add them in after cooking your food.

While protein is categorized by colour, I classify fats based on how we handle them.

Pour, cut or spread and crunch.

Fats that you pour include Omega-3's, Omega-6's and Omega-9's. You'll recognize them because they're liquid at room temperature.

Omega-3 fats are the gold stars of the 3 types, so be mindful and include at least 5 grams or 1 teaspoon minimum of them in your daily meal plan. They have been proven to boost immunity, are imperative for cognitive development and learning, are anti-inflammatory and help prevent Alzheimer's, cancer, heart disease, mental illness and more.

In short, they are non-negotiable if you want to have optimal health beyond weight loss.

Fish, flax, walnut, hemp and pumpkin oil -- all of which you pour -- are examples of Omega-3 fats. Omega-6 fats you pour include safflower, sesame and sunflower oil while Omega-9's are olive, avocado, peanut and almond oil.

In Western diets, the ratio of Omega-6's to Omega-3's should be about 3 to 1 or 2 to 1. Unfortunately, with all the processed crap that's found its way into our meals and snacks, you probably average a ratio of more like 40 to 1.

Another example of when good things go horribly wrong.

Our over-consumption of Omega 6's has increased inflammation in our bodies, which in turn has lead to the increased risk of cancer, diabetes, skin conditions, heart disease, arthritis, ADHD, autoimmune disease and depression. Nothing anyone wants!

Going back a few generations, many of us had to take cod liver oil off a spoon. But nowadays, we don't put anything in our mouths that doesn't taste good, which is a main cause of that Omega fats imbalance.

Back in the day, nutrition was simple. We intuitively knew what we needed to be healthy. But with our taste buds being hijacked daily, we've forgotten how to tune in and listen to our body's needs.

Just like protein, healthy fats work wonders for our circulatory system, which is another reason they are the second layer of your blueprint. A 3 to 1 or 2 to 1 ratio of Omega-6 to Omega-3 affects our cholesterol levels.

Omega-3's lower the levels of low-density lipoprotein (LDL) cholesterol -- "bad" cholesterol -- while supporting your levels of high-density lipoprotein (HDL) cho-lesterol -- "good" cholesterol. Clearly, anyone suffering from high cholesterol should add more Omega-3's into their diet, pronto!

Sometimes, changing up your meal plans means you don't have to take those medications to correct problems. You can deal with them from a nutritional standpoint.

Working with a meal plan is my favorite way to teach clients how to introduce more Omega-3's into the body. Like I mentioned earlier, many protein-rich foods contain healthy fats as well.

Salmon and avocados are perfect examples of fats that you cut. Salmon is a medium protein and counts to-wards your Omega-3 fat for the day!

The last of the 3 categories of fat is the most popular, especially among women. These are the fats we spread or crunch, such as almond butter, peanut butter, cashew butter, raw nuts and seeds, coconut oil, coconut manna and coconut flakes.

To keep the E.A.T! Framework as straightforward as possible, aim for 20 grams of fat daily -- the same num-ber as your proteins. Just make sure you get 5 of those 20 grams from the pour category, so fish oil or flaxseed oil.

Here's a few examples of what this looks like:

- 8 almonds = 5 grams of fat

- 2 walnuts = 5 grams of fat

- ¼ cup avocado = 10 grams of fat

POUR

- *Omega-3: Fish Oil, Flax Oil, Hemp Oil, Pumpkin Oil and Walnut Oil*

- *Omega-9: Olive Oil, Avocado Oil, Peanut Oil and Almond Oil*

- *Omega-6: Safflower Oil, Sunflower Oil and Sesame Oil*

CUT

- *Omega-3: Salmon (Wild) and Avocado*

SPREAD OR CRUNCH

- *Omega-3: Almond butter, peanut butter, cashew butter, raw nuts and seeds, coconut oil, coconut manna and coconut flakes*

Chapter 11
Your Nutritional Blueprint: Carbohydrates

We love to love 'em, we love to hate 'em.

CARBS.

I have never worked with a client whose emotional eating struggles did *not* revolve around excess carb intake. And I've never heard a client verbally beat themselves up because they ate too much chicken or fish!

"I was at a friend's house, and there was this dish of mini chocolate bars. . ."

"The buffet at my husband's work event had the crunchiest french fries, and one plate didn't seem like enough. . ."

"You don't understand! The dinner rolls came with a sweet buttery sauce. . ."

Hearing my clients confess their past diet "sins" is almost a religious experience.

And it's always carbohydrates that tempt us to fall.

The secret to change both your mindset and your meals is to focus all your energy not on fighting the old ways of doing and thinking, but on building the new.

If that struggle is real, the E.A.T! Framework is the right place for you. Because once you create new patterns around carb consumption, you can see the most dramatic body composition change of your life -- and even *prolong* it.

Four years ago, my client David approached me about his blood sugar problems. At 265 pounds, David pricked himself several times a day to manage diabetes. Synthetic insulin shots accompanied them, of course.

But 5 months into reworking his meals to include fewer simple carbohydrates and the right amount of proteins and fats, he dropped 25 pounds.

And that wasn't all. In David's own words, he now enjoys, ". . .excellent blood sugar levels and rarely need my insulin. I did it by changing my behaviour when it came to food. Today I feel great, have more energy, better sleep and no aches and pains during the day."

Change your carbs, change your life.

One of the keys for David -- and for most of my middle aged clients -- is getting honest with yourself about wheat.

It's the ultimate appetite stimulant and contains more sugar than sugar itself after your body digests it.

But E.A.T! isn't about banning any one food, even wheat, unless you're sensitive to gluten. It's about choosing foods that support the person you want to become. If you're trying to lose weight, why would you eat something that's going to stimulate your appetite?

Now, having said that, a wave of wheat-free and gluten-free foods has overtaken grocery stores all across North America. The fad reminds me of the Atkins diet era, when low-carb foods rocked every shelf wherever groceries were sold.

This probably comes as no surprise to you -- the low-carb foods didn't necessarily make you feel your best. In fact, many of them made you feel incredibly bloated and gassy!

The same thing is going on with the gluten-free food phenomenon. Just because it's gluten-free does not mean it's good for you. Corn starch, rice starch, potato starch and tapioca starch are all powerful carbohydrates that manipulate your body composition.

Gluten-free just isn't a synonym for weight loss; that's not how it works. Gluten-free products are designed to give options to people who have serious illnesses such as IBS, Crohn's and Celiac. Even then, I still recommend clients stay away from these products. If your body is rejecting processed foods, the solution isn't to find processed alternatives.

To continue this long overdue rant about the power of carbohydrates, they also impact your mood and disrupt your sleep patterns. Thanks to all the sugar in refined carbohydrates, including whole wheat bread, your body experiences spikes in insulin levels, which cause belly fat, elevate your stress hormones and lead to metabolic syndrome.

The bottom line with any refined carbohydrates is that they're not a friend of your overall health. They're more like that first college roommate you had a lot of fun with at late-night weekend parties, but her influence led directly to poor grades that semester.

I want you to feel great all day long. To have energy for your workouts, to chase your kids and to take on all the challenges of daily life.

The goal is to always feel full and satisfied and not like your head's going to drop on the desk at 3 in the afternoon. You CAN change your body composition by managing your carbohydrates and the powerful insulin spikes they cause. It's just a matter of changing up the type of carbohydrates and the portions you're eating, to support not having those spikes in blood sugar levels.

We'll get to the 2 types of carbs in a few paragraphs. For now, let's end the rant with another healthy dose of truth.

The food you eat can either be the safest and most powerful form of medicine, or the slowest and most potent form of poison.

Your choice.

At the end of the day -- literally! -- most women only need 25 grams of complex carbohydrates per serving, 3 servings per day. In fact, make that your *maximum* unless you're a super-active athlete.

Now, let me explain what 25 grams of carbohydrates looks like. This is the amount of carbohydrates contained in the serving size, NOT the weight measure of this macronutrient.

- 25 grams of potatoes is 4 oz or 1 cup serving

- 25 grams of scottish or steel cut oatmeal ½ cup serving

- 25 grams of chickpeas is 3 oz or ½ cup serving

- Silverhill's brand squirrelly bread is 1.5 slices

Take one look at those numbers, and you can also see how quickly they add up and how we can overeat them without even realizing it.

So let's dive into learning more about this powerful macronutrient so we can strip away the fear and help you learn to love AND respect carbs.

There are 2 types of carbohydrates you need to know about; simple and complex. Regardless of type, all carbohydrates need to be consumed responsibly if you want your body to look and feel great.

First, let's understand simple carbohydrates. These carbs require little to no digestion by the body, so they provide you with instant energy before conversion into glycogen or body fat. Glycogen is stored in our muscles unless we overload the body with carbs.

Think of it this way; your lean body mass is basically a big storage bin. When it gets full, there's no more room to store glycogen, so it ends up stored in your torso, belly, thighs and elsewhere as plain old body fat.

This is why finding that right balance of carbohydrates for you is so incredibly important. You want your body to convert the carbs into glycogen, then back into energy when you exercise regularly. (You're exercising regularly, right?)

We all know most of the simple carbs by name: sugar, dairy, fruit, maltose, high fructose corn syrup, honey, malt syrup, molasses and dextrose.

So how do we fit simple carbohydrates into the E.A.T! framework? Easy! We incorporate fruit.

I will never understand how or why anyone would want to eliminate this food group from their diet. It's nature's candy, and I can't imagine never tasting a sweet, ripe piece of pineapple or the crunch of a honey crisp apple again.

The rule of thumb I have my clients follow is to have 2 servings of fruit per day either as it comes packaged or about a single cup serving size. Let your tastebuds guide your choices here, but keep it to just those 2 servings.

If you've ever been on a low-fat diet where you never lost weight, now you know why. With all that fruit and yogurt you ate, how could you possibly ever drop even an inch?

Simple carbohydrates are like kindling on a campfire. You put the kindling on, see a big flame and feel a burst of heat. A few seconds later, it's gone. Burned out as quickly as it appeared. In essence, this is what simple carbohydrates do inside your body.

Complex carbohydrates, however, are the slow burning log on that camp fire. It stays hot for hours. Complex carbs are much harder for your body to break down.

Known as starches or dietary fiber, they help sustain normal blood sugar levels, help you feel full after a meal, prevent constipation and increase both fat and cholesterol absorption. They can only be found in plant based foods, including potatoes, grains, beans, peas, yam, corn, sweet potatoes, grainy breads and rice.

The most important fact I want you taking away from this tour through the world of carbohydrates is that you should not be afraid of them -- even simple carbs!

Again, you don't need to stop eating them or go all paleo. Eating in alignment with your desired body composition is all about paying attention to portion sizes. Carbs are your energy foods, so it makes sense that you eat them when you need energy, not when you're lounging on the couch at midnight on a Friday.

To ensure you're filling up your 25 grams per serving with the best carbs on the planet, let's take it one step further than simple versus complex carbs.

Whether it's with a 1-on-1 client or the group program version of the E.A.T! Framework, I work with 3 categories of carbs which I assign ratings to based on their source.

Are the carbs from the earth, a field or a box?

The earth category gets an A+ grade. You can find these type of carbohydrates grown in the earth (obviously), such as potatoes, yams, beets and turnips.

Carbs from a field earn an A- grade and include, you guessed it, carbs grown in a field! Unprocessed grains like barley and wild rice make up this category.

Then there is the box category, which gets a B rating (and makes it easy to remember). These carbohydrates are usually processed and also include any carb-rich foods found in bags, bars, bread (yes even the grainy ones) and beans.

This is the category of "healthy convenience foods", but in a perfect world, you eat no more than one serving of B carbs per day if you can avoid it.

A quick note about beans -- if you're soaking them before cooking them in their natural state, you can consider them Field category. But if you're cracking a can open to eat them, they stay in the B category.

Again, we're focusing on quality of food. Beans packed into a can loaded with sodium are NOT the best choice for your body.

And then. . .there's corn.

Corn makes things fat, *fast*. That's why factory farmers use corn as cattle feed nowadays, so baby cows grow into giant, overweight cows ready for market sooner. So enjoy it, but as with all other carbohydrates, moderating and understanding your portion size are key.

Rather than give you a to-do list for carbohydrates, I want you to simply reflect on what you're learning. From now on, pay attention to which types of carbs you usually put on your plate. You're going to have your entire life to revise your choices and get dialed into which sources of complex carbs make you feel your best.

Unlike your healthy fats, eat your carbohydrates earlier in the day. This is when we're most active. You're up with the kids, you're running around, you're exercising, you're headed to work and you need your brain and body fired up.

Like I stated above, you *do not* want to be eating these foods late in the evening while sitting in front of the TV. Number 1, your body doesn't need the energy; and number 2, some carbohydrates stimulate your hunger. You want your food to be working *for* you, to avoid late night triggers that can start a chip binge, especially if you're trying to change your body composition.

That's what I call the best of both worlds! Your food is working for you to change your body composition.

Of course, nothing bad will happen if you DO eat complex carbs at dinner -- or if it's accompanied by that flank steak right off the grill. For some, it's a real challenge to go from eating a "normal" dinner to a plate of only fibrous vegetables!

The point of all this isn't about "fixing" you, it's about learning to make the choices that best support what you want more often than not. I personally gave up eating complex carbohydrates at dinner years ago, so it's really hard for me to eat them at night now because my body just doesn't crave them anymore. If I do choose to eat them when I'm out for dinner, for example, I wake up the next morning feeling like I have a food hangover or just have a crappy sleep!

Notice how the E.A.T! Framework goes beyond weight loss and counting calories to, "How does this food impact my life?" Eating right for your body is about more than keeping 2 eyes on that scale at all times.

So whether they're A+ or A-, what do those 25 grams per serving of carbs actually look like in a real person's diet?

Keep the carbs in the earlier half of the day, for starters. Get in your 3 servings over breakfast, a mid-morning meal and at lunch.

At breakfast, toast a slice of grainy, dense bread and pair it with two hard-boiled eggs. By grainy and dense, I mean any kind of bread you can't "squish." This rules out wheat and even whole wheat. Check the nutrition label to see how many grams of carbohydrates are in a slice and adjust accordingly to meet your 25 grams.

For that mid morning meal, I like to mix Scottish cut or steel cut oats into non-fat Greek yogurt, then toss mixed berries in to top it off. It's not the fanciest, but it tastes amazing -- especially if you seal it in a mason jar overnight so the oats can absorb the moisture.

Then you can close out your carbs for the day with a serving of root vegetables alongside your chicken breast and grilled asparagus. Sprinkle black pepper on the potatoes, or cinnamon on yams.

You've probably picked up a pattern by now -- it's downright EASY to E.A.T! In fact, you might be scratching your head, feeling like something is missing. There's no calorie counter and calculator or nutrition charts that look like a multiplication table.

Proteins, fats and carbohydrates -- when you know the serving sizes to eat each day, and which foods to get those servings from, guess what happens? *You're free to just eat the damn food!* No guilt-inducing accountability or finger-wagging judgment needed.

As you implement your personalized framework for the other foods that make up a complete meal plan in the chapters ahead, I guarantee you'll see more than your body composition change. You'll sleep much deeper and more peacefully, and wake up in the morning energized and ready to go.

Snooze button, you've met your match!

PROGRESS NOT PERFECTION

Eat the complex carbohydrates that support your ideal body composition. It's easy as the three grades -- A+, A- and B. Hang out in the A's, watch out for the B's and you won't have to worry about glycogen running amok in your body.

Below, note which carbohydrates receive which grades based on their source -- the earth, a field or a box.

When log your food, pay attention to what categories you're getting most of your carbohydrates from. Stay curious, but not judgy.

EARTH CARBS (A+)

- Potatoes, sweet potatoes and yams
- Acorn squash, butternut squash, spaghetti squash and pumpkins
- Beets, turnips and parsnips
- Bananas (These count as a serving of fruit AND a complex carb.)

FIELD CARBS (A-)

- Barley
- quinoa
- millet
- wild rice
- steel-cut oats / scottish oats
- amaranth

BOX CARBS (B)

- Canned lentils and beans
- Quick Oatmeal
- Meal replacement bars, protein bars, energy bars
- Ezekiel bread and "squirrelly" bread
- Any boxed or bagged "healthy" food. (Read your labels and KNOW what you're eating.)
- Pasta (Limit this to no more than once per week. Choose rice pasta and watch your portion sizes like a hawk.)

Chapter 12
Your Nutritional Blueprint: Fruits and Vegetables

The food pyramid we all saw in school growing up, is wrong. Very, VERY wrong.

Remember the foundation? *Grains*. We're supposed to have 4 *entire* servings of grains per day and only 2 to 4 servings of fruits and veggies, according to that f-ing pyramid.

Of course, the fact that the E.A.T! Framework deviates from the official institutional recommendation shouldn't come as any surprise. I am definitely not one to echo the sentiments of the "experts" whose diet plans keep us unhappy, unfulfilled and unhealthy.

To give your body the nutrients it needs, separate your fruits and vegetables. One category is filled with carbohydrates, the other with minerals and fibre.

For the average woman, 2 servings of fruit per day is the maximum your body needs. Even if your head is filled with ideas about no-carb or slow-carb eating, I am not about to have you put in place a total ban on fruit. Remember Chapter 11?

Any fresh food consumed in moderation won't wreck your body.

And by moderation, I don't mean one of those unnaturally ginormous Fuji apples that are as big as your head. That is NOT 1 serving, okay? A single serving of fruit is the package it arrived to humanity in from the Universe, God, whatever you want to call it. It's approximately 1 cup, no more.

If you're having dried fruit, stick to ¼ cup serving if you want to avoid overeating. Dried fruit is highly concentrated because the water has been removed. It's easy to put back the sugar of 5 apples when you start munching on delicious apple chips.

That's not the only way women over-consume fruit. I see SO many women throwing chunks of fruit into their "green" smoothies and juicing fruit several times a week. *Think of all that sugar.*

Remember, just because it's healthy for you does not mean it's going to help you lose weight if you're overeating it.

So, here's how we play with fruit inside the E.A.T! Framework:

Give yourself 2 servings per day in combination with your protein and complex carb meal, or with a protein and fat rich meal.

Here are a few examples of how you can incorporate fruit. ({P} stands for protein, {F} stands for fat, {CC} stands for complex carbohydrate.)

Smoothie:

¾ cup nonfat greek yogurt {P}

1 cup frozen berries

1 cup spinach

½ cup cooked oatmeal (cooled) {CC}

Meals:

3 ounces of grilled turkey {P}

½ cup of chickpeas {CC}

1 cup blueberries

Mixed greens

2 Eggs {P}

Grilled mushrooms and asparagus

Banana {CC}

Tuna tataki {P}

Pine nuts {F}

Mixed greens

Orange slices

Nonfat Greek yogurt {P}

Flax oil {F}

Cocoa powder

Vanilla stevia

Fruit slices

E.A.T! is all about freedom, and that means your fruit is free to take whatever shape, color or texture you like. Nothing bad is going to happen if you have 3 cups of fruit in 1 day. These recipes are guidelines, not laws set in stone for all time. If you want to swirl a handful of fresh raspberries into your Greek yogurt before an evening workout at the gym, guess who *won't* be pointing a finger at you -- me.

It's always amusing when, at the end of group pro-gram version of E.A.T!, clients come to me and say, "I've been SO bad. I totally binged on this bag of raw almonds and banana chips."

I tilt my head and answer back, "Yes, but do you re-member what you were eating before you started? A whole candy bar every single day!"

Isn't it amazing (and not in a good way) that we can go from judging ourselves for eating too many Mars bars to beating ourselves up for eating too many apple chips?

Your choices are *naturally* going to become better for you the more you know what your body needs -- such as a max of 2 fruit servings a day. Let's put down the judg-ments and own those choices. Even if that means we binge on a bag of raw almonds and apple chips.

As for your veggies, let your freak flag fly! Forget that 2 to 4 servings a day shit -- aim for 9.

Yes, 9 servings of vegetables a day, preferably the leafy green kind.

"Nine servings, Lisa? Are you crazy?!" I've had clients wonder if that guideline was a misprint.

The truth is, 9 servings isn't a lot. That salad you had for lunch with the spinach and its toppings of carrots and red and green peppers -- that's 3 whole servings right there!

If you're now wondering just how on earth you're going to get in the remaining 6 cups in, dreading the thought of carrying around 3 or 4 jars of canned spinach in your purse, start simple.

Progress, not perfection.

Your body will be happy even if you only get 3 servings of leafy green veggies in per day. I know some women who gulp that down in a single kale and lime smoothie before 7 in the morning!

If vegetables have been sparse in your diet the past few years, then I definitely want you easing into the maximum of 9 servings per day. Add in 1 new serving per day. Start with the green leafy ones, then focus on choosing different colours, like white cauliflower, orange bell peppers or yellow jalapeños (if you like your veggies spicy).

Over the coming weeks, be gentle with your digestive system. If you introduce too much fibre into your diet too quickly, you can end up feeling incredibly constipated. Cooking and processing your veggies before eating them is one of the smoothest ways to add more servings without making you irregular.

And by processing, I mean a *food processor*. One of my favorite all-time recipes for a zesty triple serving of veggies is one you can eat with your favorite squirrelly bread.

Cut up an eggplant and red peppers and roast them in the oven, then toss them into the food processor or blender with a teaspoon of flax oil and a few handfuls of spinach. This makes an amazing roasted red pepper dip for veggies or a topping for chicken. You can also use it for a spread on your toasted grainy bread or brown rice crackers.

No matter how you prepare your veggies, don't be afraid to modify recipes by decreasing the amount of fat they call for or, better yet, add healthy fats like flax oil after the fact so they fit your serving numbers. Remember, flax oil is heat-sensitive so you can't cook with it. But you can easily add it to hot food after it's cooked.

Vegetables contain fat soluble vitamins, so for your body to absorb them properly, it actually makes sense to eat them with a serving of healthy fats. Animal proteins contain residual fats too, so eating a pork chop with your cauliflower will do the trick.

Giving your body everything it needs to thrive is as simple as eating a complete meal, one meal after the next. Add in 1 more veggie serving into your day when you feel adventurous, and you'll be able to tell the difference.

So, now you know -- the foundational layer of the *real* food pyramid isn't pasta, it's peppers!

PROGRESS NOT PERFECTION

Like Popeye the Sailor taught us, dark leafy green veggies strengthen our bodies. But did you also know they're rich in vitamins and minerals like folic acid, iron, potassium, B vitamins and magnesium?

Other veggies are our allies, too. One serving of broccoli contains more vitamin C than a glass of milk, and a cup of chopped peppers offers 3 times the C as a peeled orange!

Consult the list below to get your minimum of 3 leafy green veggie servings per day.

Take some time to look at your food log and see how you're doing with your fruit and veggies servings.

Are you overeating or undereating them?

Set your intentions for the week and decide which ones (and where) you're going to add to your meals.

Pick 1 veggie from the list below that you've never tried, and add it to your shopping list this week. For added points, check out my Pinterest page (Pinterest.com/LCarpenterInc) for a new and simple veggie recipe you've never tried.

YOUR LEAFY GREEN VEGGIE SHOPPING LIST:

- Kale
- Spinach
- Turnip greens

- Mustard greens
- Collard greens
- Swiss chard
- Bok choy
- Spinach
- Red and green lettuce
- Cabbage
- Arugula
- Brussel sprouts
- Mixed Greens
- Eggplant
- Carrots
- Peppers (multi-color)
- Radishes
- Cucumber
- Zucchini
- Celery
- Onion
- Artichokes
- Asparagus
- Green Beans
- Mushrooms

Chapter 13
Your Nutritional Blueprint: Legumes

Let's talk about beans.

Depending on which health blogs you read or fitness magazines you subscribe to, legumes are the wonder food of weight loss.

What does the typical consumer do then when faced with overwhelming support for an alleged "health" food? Write it on the shopping list, throw it in your cart and tear into it that evening for dinner like it's going to give you immortality!

And what gets completely ignored in this scenario?

The label.

In a world where weightlifters and fitness instructors brag about how many cans of beans they consume per day, we owe it to our bodies to peer behind the hype.

That means reading the damn label.

And when you do, you'll find that beans and lentils aren't that perfect protein source they're cracked up to be.

A cup of boiled lentil beans contains 17 grams of protein. Cool, right?

Except. . .*no*. That same serving brings with it 40 grams of carbohydrates -- almost double the recommended serving size for a complex carbohydrate!

Kidney beans and quinoa are about the same, except they offer even fewer grams of protein per carb-rich serving.

Only edamame is almost equal parts protein to complex carbs and will count as a full protein and complex carb meal.

The point of me exposing the true carb count of beans and legumes is not so you'll dump them in the trash or leave them rotting in the back of the fridge. I want all of my clients to feel confident in the choices they're making as they push the cart around the grocery store.

Just because foods have a reputation, doesn't mean the reputation is accurate. Legumes are one of the biggest offenders. The truth is, they don't offer near enough protein to warrant consideration as a full protein serving. This means that if you *did* eat enough beans to reach a full serving, you would exceed the volume of complex carbohydrates your body needs.

Peanuts are another offender worth mentioning. As part of the legume family, they're often used as a protein source. In my recipes I treat peanuts as a source of fats -- NOT protein. Although in a small ¼ cup serving you'll find an impressive 9 grams of protein, you'll also be consuming over 18 grams of fat. If you remember my pointers in Chapter 10, you know that's almost the entire amount of healthy fat E.A.T! recommends for an entire day!

This is exactly why people who eat a plant-based diets wrestle with their body composition. They consume way too many damn fats (and carbs)! I've already stated I'm a huge fan of animal based protein. However, if you are plant based and that's not an option, you must still monitor the volume of complex carbs you're eating. You can find many plant based protein supplements on the market now to help you increase your protein intake without increasing your waist size or compromising your values.

All you have to do is read the label to learn the truth. Food manufacturers deceive us with misleading information like, "Get 17 grams of protein per serving!" Of course, they neglect to mention the fact that "1" serving size of those beans offers *double* the carbs your body needs per serving.

What looks like protein is usually a complex carbohydrate. Again, manufacturers just want us to buy what they're selling, whether it's a healthy or refined food. It's still a business. So it's your responsibility as a consumer to have the courage to read labels and get savvy. You must look at the serving size and numbers for every macronutrient before you assume a food is high in anything.

Ask yourself, "How long is this list of ingredients? Where does sugar show up? Is this something I even want to put in my body? If not, why would I be willing to put it into my kids' bodies?"

That's the thing about our children. Quite often, we overfeed them by a long shot. Kids instinctively know how to graze. They eat when they're hungry, and they don't eat when they're not hungry. Any parent knows the frustration around this. So, feed them more often and keep their serving size smaller.

If you're buying a nutritionally dense bread ·· 1 piece of bread, half a sandwich ·· is plenty for your little munchkin. They can have the other half later. Two slices of bread is closer to a serving size for an adult, by the way.

To keep this as straightforward as possible, whether you're shopping for your breakfast or for baby, remember that short ingredients lists are good; long lists are not.

If there are more carbs or fat than protein, it doesn't count as protein.

Simple guidelines, easy results. That's how you E.A.T!

PROGRESS NOT PERFECTION

Many "healthy" food products can sabotage our journey to ideal body composition if we don't read the labels. Be mindful of the list below so you don't fall prey to manipulative food manufacturers!

READING A FOOD LABEL (SO A SERVING OF PROTEIN DOESN'T BECOME TWO SERVINGS OF CARBS)

1. What is the serving size listed on the label?

2. What is the ratio of protein to carbohydrates?

3. What does the serving size look like to fit into your E.A.T! guidelines?

4. How many grams of protein and complex carbohydrates are in your adjusted E.A.T! serving size?

Chapter 14
Your Nutritional Blueprint: Mayo, Milk and Merlot

No nutritional blueprint is complete if all you can have for lunch is a chicken breast sandwich on plain Ezekiel bread with half an apple and a tossed salad minus the dressing.

What a bland world that would be to live in -- and eat in!

As this chapter's title reveals, we've got to take a good look at condiments, dairy and alcohol and the role they play in a well balanced diet that supports an ideal body composition.

The truth is, if eating well isn't an adventure for your tastebuds, you're going to quit. Period. I've seen it happen a thousand times. Deprivation *always* leads to weight gain. And that's not what you're here for.

Because of that, condiments are a crucial aspect of your nutritional blueprint to liven up every meal.

Now, I'm not the kind of girl who likes to hang out in the kitchen for hours at a time. So I'm okay with the fact that I don't make my mayo from scratch. You should be, too. I prefer quick and easy with minimal prep time.

That means I always make sure my plain organic beef, chicken breast and hard-boiled eggs -- all the staples -- are waiting for me in the fridge throughout the week. (See the specifics of meal planning in Chapter 15.)

I do want to note that just because I eat organic, doesn't mean you need to. Start where you're at, and remember that healthy eating is an evolution. I just want you to eat protein, for example, so don't get caught up in much more than that when you're starting out.

Depending on whatever specific flavor I'm feeling on a given day, I can add a dash of spices or a dollop of sauce to my protein and veggies.

When it comes to condiments, there has been a big push to eliminate sugar from meals entirely. I totally get that. However, I'm also 100% percent in support of your food actually tasting good!

So, what's a reasonable condiment?

Remember our go-to move from Chapter 13?

Always check that label.

A 1 teaspoon serving size that has 30 grams of carbohydrates is just not reasonable.

Pad Thai sauce is especially popular here in Canada, but we have to be mindful of the fact that sugar is the main ingredient.

Again, rather than toss it into the garbage, let's be respectful. Sugary condiments are not evil as long as we commit to consumption in moderation. A teaspoon goes a long way, so measure carefully. Condiments are not free-pour territory!

But rather than calorie-counting, it sometimes make sense to simply choose a different condiment that still offers flavour. For example, spread apple butter on your Ezekiel bread instead of jam. In 1 tablespoon, you find only 4 grams of carbohydrates. That's quite a serving for so few carbs! Mix it in with your Greek yogurt, and you have a delicious dairy delight.

I just think it's unreasonable to assume we can go through this entire lifetime without consuming any sugar. So if enjoying your Pad Thai sauce means you're going to eat healthier longer because your food isn't plain and boring, go for it.

And even though we need those fats, check the condiment labels carefully for them, too. Every serving size should contain 5 grams or less of fat.

Those salty condiments are absolute must-haves for a complete flavor experience, too. It's easy to have ground turkey in the fridge and then mix a little bit of hoisin sauce and water in with a few peanuts and a handful of lettuce.

While I like my mustards, they are high in sodium, so take caution especially with your salad dressings. Normal daily intake for sodium is about 1300 to 1500 milligrams. Don't shy away from the salt, as low sodium is just as bad for your health as high sodium. So whenever you're missing that salt kick, add a dash of Himalayan sea salt to your salad at dinner to give your body what it needs.

The healthier you eat, the less you need to worry about over-consuming sodium. For most, it's only a problem when you're consuming a diet overrun by processed foods.

Honestly, if they took the sodium out of processed food, we wouldn't have an obesity problem! Salt, just like fat, makes food taste good, which hijacks our tastebuds.

Watching your sodium intake is particularly important if you struggle with high blood pressure. Fortunately, when you change how you're eating and remain mindful of those saltier foods, high blood pressure can become a thing of the past.

No matter what condiments have been your go-to's in the past, they are bound to start getting "old" as you build out your nutritional blueprint with all those proteins and veggies.

That's why I advise clients to get creative and, yes, *play with their food*! If you don't like a new condiment, never buy it again. But at least have the courage to try.

One of my favorite weird condiment creations is avocado, horseradish and sweet chili sauce together with either bok choy or brussel sprouts and ground beef, chicken or turkey.

Dozens of different meal combinations from just 8 foods! Who knew amazing varieties could be so easy?

I did briefly mention yogurt a few paragraphs ago, so let's not get any further on this flavour train without addressing dairy.

"Lisa, isn't cheese a protein? How much of it can I eat? I freaking LOVE cheese."

This question comes at me on the first call of every group program I run. My answer is always the same.

No.

Cheese does not count as a protein. With it, we run into the same problem as legumes. Yes, there's protein there, but most cheeses contain more fat than you will ever find in real protein. In fact, in a quarter cup serving of medium aged cheddar, you get 11 grams of fat and only 7 grams of protein.

The rule of thumb for both fat and protein is that 1 gram of fat is 9 calories, whereas 1 gram of protein is only 4. Do the math on cheese, and you're getting WAY too much of what your body doesn't need for every gram of protein you do.

Just like certain condiments, another problem with cheese is the sodium. If you took out the salt, cheese would taste as plain as a napkin. That's why it is so easy to have a single bite of cheese from the party tray. . .then another. . .then another. . .then another 'til all the pepper jack is gone and you don't even realize where it went.

If you do choose to eat cheese, treat it the same way you would a decadent dessert. Eat it in moderation, and eat it consciously. I love blue cheese on my steak, but only on occasion. Cheese is NOT a staple in my everyday diet.

When it comes to that other popular dairy product ·· milk ·· always choose skim or 1% and use it in moderation. I treat milk more as a condiment than a protein, and that makes sense for my clients, too.

Thanks to the low fat trend from years past, low fat milk has become popular. However, sales of full fat dairy products are up, too.

Why? Because we love our fatty, milk and cheese! Food manufacturers moved the fat from milk and increased production of full fat cheese.

Food producers ALWAYS have their eye on their bottom line, not on our overall health and wellbeing. Waste is not profitable.

Dairy can also be a digestive nightmare for certain people. Every Naturopathic Doctor I've met will steer you clear of it. It's worth paying attention to how your body feels eating dairy, but again, you must feel your way into this instead of just eliminating something because of someone else's opinion. Nevertheless, it's been the proven culprit behind digestive issues, IBS, bloating and more.

Start implementing the E.A.T! Framework, and once you feel confident in all the components, you can start testing to see what is and is not agreeing with your body.

If you're curious if milk, cheese, condiments or any other foods are giving you discomfort, take them out of your meal plan for a week. Then see what happens. Do you feel better? Do you feel worse?

Add a category back in one at a time so you can identify the culprit quickly. With the knowledge you have from

E.A.T!, your version of an elimination diet is as simple as checking one box off at a time. Did you start feeling better after taking Greek yogurt out as one of your proteins for a week? No? Move on to grains.

This works much better to ease your body's stress than doing a radical elimination diet. Besides, once you know how to E.A.T!, getting assistance from a Naturopath is easy to navigate.

The more you know, the more you can make choices that are in alignment with your ideal body composition. *And you cannot unknow what you now know.*

Which leads us to probably the most controversial category of all.

Alcohol.

I have no intention of telling you what you can or can't drink or what you should and shouldn't drink. It's 100% your choice.

What I WILL do is educate you on how alcohol impacts your weight loss intentions. Unfortunately, booze really does get in the way of shedding pounds, and that's not just because of the calories in alcohol. Calorically speaking, alcohol has 7 calories per gram whereas fat has 9. That's still a lot.

Alcohol inhibits your body's ability to burn fat. Even 1 drink of lite beer spikes your cortisol levels -- your stress hormone -- which slows down your metabolism.

So clearly, alcohol is not supportive of your best health!

But that's not the end of alcohol's baggage. It also speeds up muscle loss and impairs muscle recovery.

As women, it is imperative that we maintain our lean mass to keep that fat-burning engine running. If the size of our engine decreases, which we're already fighting as we age, we can end up gaining weight even if nothing in our diet changes.

The other thing we need to be aware of with alcohol is that it lowers our inhibitions. So if you have 1 drink at a party, the next thing you know, you're hovering over the buffet table with a slice of cake and your favourite chips!

I'm not just talking beer or spirits here. That bottle of wine after work to take the edge off your day could very well be making it worse thanks to the long term negative effects on your body.

So whether you pour a glass of cabernet every night or make your own bloody mary vodka mixes, if you haven't seen the body composition changes you hoped for, you now know why.

It may be time to decide what kind of healthy boundaries you'd like to have.

Start with 2 weeks off from alcohol, then incorporate 1 glass a week back in and see how you feel. It's not about depriving, it's about testing.

So find out, be honest with yourself and make choices that align with who you want to be.

After all. . .

It's *your* body.

PROGRESS NOT PERFECTION

If your body composition results don't match your intentions, don't get discouraged. And don't ask yourself why. *Go find out!*

To rule out why you're not feeling well -- and to identify the cause of discomfort -- eliminate each of the following foods from your diet at a time.

After 1 week without it, introduce that food back in and note any changes. Log how you feel after eating each food taking that break. Fairly quickly, you'll have the answers you seek so you can give your body what it needs.

THE TESTING NOT DEPRIVING LIST:

☐ Grains

☐ Cheese

☐ Milk

☐ Beer

☐ Wine

☐ Spirits (Vodka, etc.)

Chapter 15
Building Your Blueprint: The Ultimate Guide to Meal Planning

So, you've got your protein.

You're eating enough fats.

You're conscious of carbs.

Your meals are now a nutritious cornucopia of colours and flavours.

Yet this is exactly the point where most people fall off the wagon.

. . .if this was a diet, that is.

Eating in alignment with your ideal body composition is *easy*. . .for a few weeks.

Choosing the salad over steak isn't that hard. . .for a few meals.

But unless you KNOW you're going to enjoy the rest of your life's breakfasts, lunches and dinners, it's easy to tell your body, "No, I WON'T give you what you need. It's too hard!"

On average, we have each have about 17,000 days left on this planet. That totals up to *51,000* meals to plan! Unless you have an easy-peasy plan to make those meals nutritious, you might as well quit now.

Of course, that's why I wrote this chapter. Now that we've prepared your Nutritional Blueprint, it's time to build 1 vitamin-rich meal at a time, 1 meal after the other.

After my clients learn what they really want to eat -- and why they enjoy eating -- they ask me, "I know all the bits of pieces of eating right for me now. So how do I prep meals that have all the proteins and carbs and fats I need?"

The mindset you read about so much in the first few chapters plays a HUGE role here. Following the E.A.T! Framework is not just something you can do on a Monday or Friday.

And if you think, "If everything falls into place in my life, I'll be able to make this work, but if one thing is off I'll fall apart," then guess what? You WILL fall apart!

So before you put pen to paper to plan next week's meals, level up your consciousness.

Eating and drinking requires *thinking*.

This means you actually have to make the decision that you are going to stay conscious about food. When you go grocery shopping this week, remember what you want for yourself and how you want to feel, then make decisions from that place, from that mindset.

You're reading this book because you don't want to feel crappy anymore.

You want to feel confident and in control of your life and your body.

You want to have that sense of freedom around food.

Remember what you want.

Even though you expect progress, there WILL be days where you forgot to buy an avocado, the Pad Thai sauce is gone and the ground turkey in the back of the fridge is about as appetizing as the rotten, soggy salad next to it that you forgot about last Thursday.

When these moments happen, you'll feel the urge to say, "Screw it, I'm ordering pizza!"

It's okay to feel that. Instead of battling it out -- and, of course, ultimately losing the willpower game -- check in with yourself.

"Okay, what are my options here? I still have a few slices of Ezekiel bread left. There are salt and pepper for the turkey on the counter. I guess that doesn't sound too bad. . . Hey, I really can do this!"

In minutes, you've averted a cravings crisis that otherwise would have put an end to the hopes and dreams that motivated you to buy this book in the first place.

And what the hell, if it helps, channel yours truly if you need to!

"What would Lisa think? What Lisa would be looking for? If this was Lisa, how would she do it?"

Sometimes we have to behave our way to success. What does a successful person look like? How do they think?

This mindset isn't just for your own kitchen. Whenever I go out and about, I never roam on autopilot and feel jerked to and fro by cravings.

For example, I went into a Starbucks the other day. I hadn't had the chance to have breakfast yet because one of my sons needed to pay a visit to the doctor.

As I breathed in the fresh vanilla aroma of the 100-grams-of-sugar frappuccinos being prepared behind the counter, I kept my wits about me.

I checked in and asked myself. "Okay, what am I going to eat here?"

After surveying the selection of fatty omelettes and sugary pastries, I decided to settle on the egg white wrap with the low-fat turkey bacon.

I wasn't sure what the hell that turkey bacon thing was, but that's neither here nor there.

I made the best choice of all the options available.

I asked the barista to warm the wrap up so I could take it apart and eat only the egg white and turkey bacon because I personally don't eat any bread. I get my carbs in later on every morning.

Those are my own guidelines for *me*, not rules for *you*. That's how it should be, right?

I didn't say, I *can't* eat bread. I just don't like it!

And if there's anything I want you taking away from the E.A.T! Framework, it's that you shouldn't eat stuff you don't like. (I wish that went without saying.)

Like me, pay attention when you're out and about on your daily travels with all the options available to you to eat on the run.

Do you really want it, or is it just convenient?

At the grocery, you can buy hardboiled eggs already peeled and sealed in a package. They make do in a pinch.

Now, about that rotisserie chicken -- is that going to be the cleanest thing for you? It will be better than grabbing a chocolate bar, that's for sure!

Remember, we're not looking for perfect, we're looking for "What do I need here? I know I need a protein?" THAT is what progress is in real life. After you ask yourself, "What are my options?" move forward from there.

Fretting over each and every decision drains your willpower. There's nothing worse than eating in alignment with your body composition, then gulping half a liter of soda that night because you ran out of willpower!

The key to effective meal planning is not this fantasy where you get every gram of everything exact. Instead, plan your meals around your life. The other way around just doesn't work, trust me on that.

Ask yourself what your week looks like, the way a parent does with the kids' schedule. If you are a parent and you try to get in the perfect meal every time your kid sits down at the dinner table, you will drive yourself crazy!

Look at your own meals that way in the week ahead.

If you know you've got barbeques coming up, plan for it. If you are trying to lose weight, look at the choices you're making the rest of the week. What other things could you do to balance out the barbecue? Could you focus more on your light proteins? Could you focus more on eating carbohydrates from the earth? Where could you clean things up to support the fact that you're going to enjoy food and drink you wouldn't normally have?

Think of how the *entire* week looks instead of just, "What do I need to do right now? What do I need to do today? What do I need to do for dinner tonight?"

If a meal plan is made 2 minutes before the meal, chances are, it won't support the person you want to become. That's when portion control becomes an issue, too.

To make sure you're eating the foods that taste great *and* support your body, it takes commitment to a sustainable lifestyle. That doesn't, however, mean you need a laundry list of recipes.

Just try 1 new recipe per week, that's it! If you love it, it stays in your repertoire. If you hate it, just don't make it again -- or sub in other ingredients to make it work for your taste buds.

Eating doesn't need to be this big event or drama every time you sit down to dine. Sometimes, your meals are going to be quick and easy, and you put them together in 3 minutes flat.

As long as they taste amazing, that's what matters. Some meals you're going to go out for, and they're going to be much more of a dining experience.

And if you're a busy mom like me or a busy entrepreneur or just too busy with life in general, then go easy on yourself. The more complicated the recipe, the more resistance you'll feel.

Personally, my all-time favorite recipe is taco salad. It's the most customizable meal on the planet and can be made as a hearty lunch or light dinner.

Plus, you could literally make taco salad for everyone of your remaining 50,000 meals in life -- and still not make it the same way twice! (Yes, I've done the math.)

The *Progress Not Perfection* section at the end of this chapter has the complete recipe with potential ingredients.

Meal planning can be as simple as turning that taco salad recipe into your grocery list for the month -- stock your fridge, freezer, shelves, cupboards, countertops and pantry with all the ingredients!

Another reason I favor taco salad is the fact that you can sub in a variety of different proteins, different fats and different carbohydrates. My taco salad takes all the thinking out of it for you!

Remember, this is all about you making your life EASY.

Flexible boundaries, simple guidelines.

YOU choose the structure.

If you're worried taco salad will get old after a few days (or years), go to Pinterest and pin different recipes that look like an adventure. Feel free to use my boards for inspiration at Pinterest.ca/lcarpenterinc.

So whether you're meal planning based on my taco salad recipe or one you found online, the bottom line for sustainable meal planning is to know the base ingredients.

You've got your protein, maybe some ground turkey and lean bison. Maybe tofu or fish. Then there's the flax oil and leafy greens. Perhaps a side of quinoa in place of a grain as your complex carb serving.

It's easy to modify any recipe for your meal plan by asking questions like, "Can I add a protein to the recipe? What other proteins could I use? Can I adjust the carbs and fats to stay within my personal boundaries? What can I take out or add to make this recipe work for me throughout the day?"

That last part will be especially important in the weeks and months ahead. Remember, carbs in the morning, fats in the evening.

If this makes you tilt your head every time you read it in my book, that's okay. Most people don't know the secrets we use in figure competition to get slim fast. Like my friend Lucy said to me, "Even as a nurse I was surprised to learn the importance of when and how often I eat."

Yes, all this probably feels like a lot to be mindful of. This chapter is the "ultimate" guide to meal planning, after all!

The best way to stay on track with meal planning inside the E.A.T! Framework, I've found, is to stay ahead. Food prep for the week every Sunday has been my ritual for nearly *15 years* now.

Like I said, I'm a busy gal! I don't have a ton of time to head into the kitchen and prepare fancy meals. So meal prep for me is literally making sure that my fridge is stocked with foods that support how I want to feel during the week.

If it's not, I head to the grocery to get them. Then I spend a couple of hours in the afternoon cooking my chicken breasts, grilling salmon and boiling eggs to stock the fridge with protein. With all these varieties, I can literally mix and match my meals however I like.

When it comes to the veggies, I prefer to buy mine already washed and cut up so they're ready. Again, I can just grab and go.

You are more than welcome to go the route of making big, fancy meals, but it just doesn't work for me. I really like knowing what's cooked and ready in the fridge so I can just grab it when I need it.

Food prep, therefore, is no nuisance for me. It makes the week ahead easier, so I even look forward to it. It's my few hours of self-care every Sunday. I put on some music, get the stovetop burners ready and remind myself that a small amount of labour now will free up mental bandwidth throughout the week ahead.

Self-care begins in the kitchen. I honour it as such. It's the perfect environment to listen to an audiobook and relax into the importance of making *me* a priority in my own life.

It's not inconvenient to put the time into taking care of myself. If you do view this as a time suck, I challenge you to explore your beliefs and do some journalling around this.

Whatever you do with food or meal prep or meal planning, do it from a place of love.

And don't silently agree with me 11 months of the year and forget it every December! Whether you celebrate Christmas or Hanukkah or whatever, the holidays can throw a sugary, fatty wrench into meal planning ·· if we take ourselves too seriously.

One previous Christmas a few years ago, my friend Cris decided that she would focus on loving herself, not depriving herself, when it came to holiday food. I told her that it would be okay if the scale increased a few pounds.

Guess what happened.

She came back to me that January and reported, "During the latest holiday season, I lost quite a few pounds, and the transformation has hit me more than my physical presence. I feel confident, beautiful and strong. I feel 'awake' and bigger than life. Bring it on, world."

Bring it on, world.

Say that to yourself the next time you plan a meal.

. . .on a Sunday, that is!

PROGRESS NOT PERFECTION

My all-time favorite recipe that follows the E.A.T! Framework is taco salad. You can swap in or out just about any meat, fat, veggie, fruit or grain you like and still end up with the most appetizing meal of your life.

Turn the recipe below into your shopping list for the week.

E.A.T! TACO SALAD

Protein:

- Chicken (breast or ground)
- Beef (strips or ground)
- Bison (strips or ground)
- Fish (white)
- Turkey (breast or ground)
- Chicken (thighs or dark meat)

Complex Carbs:

- Brown Rice
- Yams
- Quinoa
- Barley
- Beans
- Lentils
- Rye crackers
- Wraps

Healthy Fats:

- Flax Oil
- Avocado
- Olive Oil
- Walnut Oil

Base Ingredients:

- ½ cup natural organic non fat yogurt
- ½ cup salsa (peach pineapple, hot, medium, mango)
- Low sodium taco seasoning or fajita seasoning (can be omitted)
- Lime juice (optional)
- Hot Sauce (optional)

Mix all ingredients together and enjoy. The possibilities and tastes are endless!

Chapter 16
E.A.T!-ing Right Long Term

Success.

It's a scary word. Because it's hard.

"Success" brings up memories of every time we've failed.

Success and failure.

Good and bad.

Praise and shame.

Healthy or unhealthy.

Fit or fat.

This kind of black-or-white thinking is the norm in the diet industry. You're either a complete success or a total failure.

You look down and see the "right" number on the scale, or you don't.

It's disgusting, really. Women come to me after *decades* of trying all the eating programs you can find on the top 10 pages of Google search results.

They just don't work.

Because once they start to implement the calorie-counting or carb-cutting, the success fairies come along. They tap you on the shoulder and say, "You're officially dieting now. You have no choice but to lose weight to be successful. Or else. . .you're nothing but a failure."

I hate the success fairies.

Because success isn't a number. It's not a 1-time event. It's not an achievement.

Success is a mindset.

True success -- the kind you can experience everyday with E.A.T! -- is yours when you decide *for yourself* what success means to you.

The phrase, "I won't be successful until. . ." has no place in your vocabulary when you're in charge of your own definition of success.

That's true for our health, and it's true for all areas of life.

During my first decade in business as a Coach, I kept success at arms reach. I told myself I would be successful when I reached X number of dollars in the bank or when my debt was paid off.

I don't know where I picked up the belief that success was defined by money, but that was my only marker for years. This belief kept me from exploring my own personalized version of success beyond just the measure of money.

I'd already built out multiple group programs, worked with thousands of women, ran multiple studios, enjoyed successful online product launches and had a loving hand in changing countless women's lives through all of it.

But none of these amounted to a hill of beans because they weren't how I measured success. I was only willing to measure based on debt and my bank account.

I still remember the moment I realized what bullshit this was. I was on a live coaching call with my E.A.T! group, and I was explaining the importance of using more than the scale to define success.

Lightbulb moment.

From that second forward, I claimed success in my business, and I've never looked back.

What makes the story even more powerful is that the money followed my shift in mindset.

Our outside world is a reflection of our inner beliefs.

Take my client Tara, for example. In 7 months, Tara lost over 10 pounds and dropped 2 dress sizes and over 20 inches because she was able to change her beliefs about her body, weight loss and healthy eating.

"I quickly realized that it wasn't about the food. It was about what was underneath the food — the emotions, beliefs, and stories that were driving patterns of behavior that kept me from losing weight and ultimately being the healthiest version of myself."

The first step I took to shift my success mindset was to stop focusing on my bank account and my debt. There's a difference between being mindful of profit and loss statements, and turning every transaction into an obsession.

The second step was to repeat to myself, "I am successful," every day. I even wrote it on my bathroom mirror so I could claim it every morning and night as I brushed my teeth. I was determined to anchor in this new belief and reframe how I defined success.

The first step for you as you implement the E.A.T! Framework may be the diet equivalent of my checking account balance -- the scale.

So many of my clients define their success based on the number on that scale. Unless they've lost 30, 20, even 5 pounds, they "failed."

The truth is, E.A.T!-ing right for your ideal body composition is a learning process. Success can't only be defined by the number on the scale.

It's about how you look at food differently.

It's about feeling differently about your body.

It's about the words and phrases you use in your inner and outer dialogue.

It's about how you're putting the pieces together.

It's about how you're not reaching for candy bars as often anymore.

It's about the fact that you don't feel guilty about your choices.

There's a whole bunch of ways that you can define success as you're creating big changes in your life. If we're always looking at ONE holy metric of success -- the bank account or the scale -- we rob ourselves of the growth, change and expansion right in front of us. We're not letting ourselves see how far we've come or how much we've evolved -- and how we're still growing, learning and changing.

Success is less about the final destination and more about the journey on our way to wherever it is we're wanting to go. Every diet out there makes us believe that when we get there, we'll be happy. But the truth is, it's the *journey* that offers the most fulfilment.

Take a peek at the ingredients labels the next time you're at the grocery.

Grill chicken breasts on Sunday for an entire week's worth of lunches.

Sample new sauces and spices to give your E.A.T! Taco Salad new flavours.

Realize that you feel comfortable in your body.

No longer beat yourself up for the piece of cake you had after dinner.

Be KIND to yourself more often than not and allow yourself grace and empathy along the journey -- like my client Yvonne, who shared with me that she's feeling comfortable in her body even though she hasn't lost all her weight yet.

That's the reason I started writing (and finally finished) this book -- it's a loving wakeup call to women that *we* are in charge of what success looks like for *our own bodies*.

Let's celebrate each little victory, every moment of joy in this journey.

Embrace every meal ahead. Embrace every snack. Embrace every choice.

Your journey doesn't have to be one of struggle, where you don't believe you can trust yourself and the choices you might make. The E.A.T! Framework is all about letting go of this struggle -- giving it up completely -- so you can move forward.

Think about it. *If you gave up the struggle, what else could be possible?*

This quote sums it up:

"Don't miss out on 95% of your life to weigh 5% less."

Don't rob yourself of the opportunity to live a Full Frontal Life™.

All over social media, people vent about their diet struggles and negative body image feelings with the hashtag "#TheStruggleIsReal".

But with the E.A.T! Framework, you're empowered to counter that with your very own truth -- "#TheStruggleIsOver".

Every day, show up and what what you need to do to help move you forward. Come from that place of peace and trust.

Believe in yourself.

Doing so is like exercising a muscle. As you savor those 3 servings of leafy green veggies every day, it'll come naturally for you to start craving veggies when they're not on your plate. I've seen this happen time and time again with clients and with myself. I never thought I could be a veggie lover until I became one.

The sooner you make the choices that are *most consistent* with your ideal body composition, the better.

But let me ask you something -- even if it takes longer to get there than you'd like, are you willing to continue moving forward with grace and ease?

Are you willing to keep going even when the discomfort of following a new path creates resistance ?

For example, as much as I'd like to be able to crank out 4 or 5 live videos per day to promote my business, I've learned that doing less but doing it *better* is the sustainable way to grow my business and keep my other priorities in check.

Getting "there" faster by trying to do more (or by trying to do things perfectly) isn't a solution for sustainable business success, and it's not the solution for sustainable weight loss and lifestyle changes.

Is the daily effort and intention I put in still worth it, and will I still get "there"?
I know my answer.

But do you know yours?

However you define success and whether you experience it or not WILL come down to your choice to define it beyond just weight and your willingness to persevere. . .or not to.

The journey *must* be worth it for you, even when you don't know how long it's going to take.

That's why I keep the E.A.T! Framework so simple. The easier it is mentally to keep track of what you need to eat to reach your ideal body composition, the easier it is *emo-*

tionally. Remember, we're no longer relying on willpower but on attention and intention.

This means you'll stay in the game -- long enough to *win*. Whatever that looks like for you.

Soon, your choices will becomes habits. But it will take time to integrate E.A.T! into your lifestyle, so just remember that whatever pace you find yourself moving at, it's the right pace for you.

Three months after my client Joanne finished the live group version of E.A.T!, she "got" this concept.

"What you do along the way is just as important as getting to the end," she said.

Over time, Joanne has come to realize that, in reality, there is no end. You're never going to be done. Like I wrote in the Introduction, you're going to eat until the day you die.

There will be resistance -- if you haven't faced it already, that is! There always, always, *always* is during journeys that matter.

And I want you to embrace it!

So when you're staring at that dinner salad but your cravings are used to steak and potatoes, the mental gremlins will scream at each other inside your head.

"Oh my god! This is just like a diet! This is so much work! This is too hard!"

If quieting them for now means adding to your meal the thing you really want (but honouring the portion size), so be it.

Progress, not perfection.

Over time, as the gremlins realize that you're not out to deprive yourself (or them), their voices will fall quiet.

One day, they'll be barely a whisper.

Until then, recognize that resistance is not a negative thing. It just shows that you're stepping onto new ground.

You're creating a new normal and claiming new territory for yourself. You're breaking patterns that didn't align with how you want to look and feel, and it's just plain uncomfortable. I get that.

Change by definition means to become different, transformed or altered. Until we can be with the discomfort of change and navigate all the feels, we'll stay comfortably uncomfortable in the land of familiar.

Who wants to live there?

Resistance can also come from familiar *relationships* -- otherwise known as saboteurs.

The sooner you have a conversation with friends and family about the E.A.T! Framework that you're working into your lifestyle, the better off you (and your waistline) will be.

But you will NOT use the "d-word."

Diet.

Because that's not what E.A.T! is.

As soon as people hear "diet," they hear "deprived." And as soon as they hear "deprived," they think it's their job to save you.

If you've ever experienced the camaraderie of dieting with others, release that familiar pattern from your lifestyle. When you've dieted with girlfriends in the past, how often did it turn into a self-hate fest?

"I don't like my body. . . My pants don't fit. . . You should stop eating this and that and all those other things. . ."

As women, part of breaking the diet cycle is no longer having these conversations. Self-sabotage like this doesn't align with the success you desire -- so release it.

Instead, tell yourself, "You know what? I don't need to talk about this stuff anymore. I'm no longer okay with criticizing my body, and I feel really good about my choices. I am empowered to make the choices that are going to be best for me."

Set loving boundaries with your friends about what you're no longer available to talk about. Say no to topics that involve body bashing and food shaming.

To earn the respect of friends and family for your choice to implement the E.A.T! Framework, your key is going to be consistency.

Making the right choices for you. Over and over.

When you don't take shit from anyone, they'll stop giving it.

You must stop using your kids, your husband or even your best friend as the excuse for why you can't change your lifestyle. Unless they are sitting on you and force-feeding you, YOU are always in the driver's seat of your choices.

When I go out to eat with people, I don't get hounded for not having a glass of wine or ordering a slice of cake.

"Oh, just come on, it's only one piece," says no one to me. *Ever.*

Why do you think that is? Because I've been so consistent over the years, my family and friends respect my boundaries.

I've taken my power back.

This journey takes consistency.

Stay consistent, and success is yours -- the way *you* define it.

PROGRESS NOT PERFECTION

The choice to persevere so that you eat in alignment with how you want to look and feel week after week, month after month, requires celebration. *Consistent* celebration.

For my clients, I require them to write daily in a Victory Journal. That boost of inspiration we all want is as simple as jotting down answers to one question:

What things did you do today that helped you feel good?

Maybe you didn't beat yourself up because you chose to have a cookie. Maybe you didn't have the cookie, so you're celebrating up. Maybe you got out and moved more. Maybe you just made your choice and there was no guilt associated to it. Maybe looked yourself in the mirror and said, "Wow! I really look and feel amazing today." Maybe the fact that you even looked yourself in the eyes in the mirror is something to celebrate.

Documenting all these victories is just as important as creating them in the first place.

REDEFINE SUCCESS WITH A VICTORY JOURNAL

What things did you do today that helped you feel good?

What things did you do today that helped you feel good?

What things did you do today that helped you feel good?

What things did you do today that helped you feel good?

What things did you do today that helped you feel good?

Conclusion

"So. . . Now what?"

That's the loaded question my clients ask after I teach them how to change their relationship with their bodies, food, what the E.A.T! Framework consists of and how to makes choices that align with their ideal body composition.

Of course, they *know* the answer -- I've just spent 6 weeks showing them!

But really, the uncertainty is worry -- worry that they won't be able to "make it work," that they'll give up and go back to struggling, suffering and feeling consumed by cravings.

I'll tell you now what I always tell them:

This information is never going to go away.

You've bought this book so all the tips, techniques and tactics are yours for the keeping. Think of it like a learning aid -- come back to whichever chapter or chapters are relevant to you whenever you like.

Get your proteins ingrained again.

Get your fats ingrained again.

Get your carbohydrates ingrained again.

Slow things down, and remember -- less is more when you're working towards creating lasting habits.

Commitment to choices that lead to your ideal body composition is not a one-time, one-off event. It's a daily activity. And for many clients (and now readers), commitment is the difference between a thriving life and an untimely end to it.

After showing my friend Kent how to adjust what he ate for each meal (thanks to E.A.T!), he told me, "I easily added ten years to my life."

Another client, Bill, thanked me being there to help him make that daily commitment.

"Doing it myself was endangering my health," he said.

Maybe I really should have titled this *The Last Diet Book You'll Ever Need*!

The daily commitment I taught Kent and Bill is available to you, too.

All it takes is one choice at a time.

One meal at a time.

One day at a time.

You can make that choice.

I believe in you.

Now, it's your turn.

Believe in you, too.

PROGRESS NOT PERFECTION

If you're worried about falling off the wagon without having someone there to gently pull you in the right direction, there are several opportunities for you and I to make progress toward your ideal body composition, into a *habit for life.*

Check out the list below, and our journey together can continue!

Want more (free) resources to apply what you learned in this book?

Learn more about the book bonuses at LisaCarpenter.ca/Book

Want more support for transforming your relationship with food and your body?

Learn more about *Feelings & Food* at LisaCarpenter.ca/FF

Want to go deeper into E.A.T! with over 10 weeks of video lessons, in depth training, nutrition charts, recipes, and guides to heal your relationship with food and take back your waistline?

Learn more about *E.A.T! : Education Transformation Action* at LisaCarpenter.ca/EAT

Want one-on-one coaching to make E.A.T! stick for life?

Learn more about working 1:1 towards your definition of success at LisaCarpenter.ca

About the Author

Lisa Carpenter, CNC, CSNC, PN1, CPT, is a nutrition and life coach who empowers driven achievers to connect deeply with their emotions, free themselves from judgment, and create lasting physical and emotional transformation. With almost two decades of experience as a health and fitness professional, Lisa is a sought-after speaker, coach, and educator who helps women make peace with their bodies and free themselves from the constraints of traditional dieting.

Made in the USA
San Bernardino, CA
22 January 2020

63489150R00102